Body Building

The Definitive Manual On Fat Incineration, Muscle Development, And Holistic Well-being

(The Superlative 30-day Exercise Program Tailored For Novices)

Lionel Ford

TABLE OF CONTENT

Strategies Employed By Iconic Figures In Training And Exercise

The annals of history bear witness to the clandestine training strategies employed by celebrated bodybuilding icons, namely Eugen Sandow, Arnold Schwarzenegger, Ronnie Coleman, and Jay Cutler. The concise concepts shared herein outline a number of clandestine exercise techniques employed by esteemed icons within the realm of bodybuilding, individuals who have wholeheartedly committed themselves to attaining greatness."

Attain a more streamlined physique initially

Expend as many calories as possible during initial stages to achieve a lean physique and a well-sculpted body. An appropriate training regimen is essential for the development and maintenance of muscular strength. A significant proportion of the renowned professional bodybuilders shared a common training technique. In accordance with the esteemed traditions of bodybuilding, it is widely believed that engaging in weight training of high intensity, for three sessions per week on non-consecutive days, proves highly effective in the formation of substantial, well-defined musculature and a more toned physique.

Incorporate a limited number of isolation exercises into your routine and emphasize compound movements such as pull ups, lat pull downs, squats, Romanian deadlifts, bench press, dips, shoulder press, cable back rows, and barbell back rows.

CARDIO

Engaging in appropriate cardiovascular exercise can assist you in attaining a slender physique adorned with clearly delineated musculature. It is recommended to place greater emphasis on shorter high-intensity sessions rather than longer low-intensity sessions towards the end of weight lifting days or on rest days in order to achieve desired outcomes within a shorter timeframe.

It is advisable to prioritize the development of larger muscle groups before focusing on smaller ones.

All esteemed individuals of great renown maintained the belief that it is of utmost importance to prioritize the training of larger muscle groups over the smaller ones. Presently, in fitness facilities, one may observe a considerable number of young individuals engaging in a training method characterized by dynamic and non-linear movements known as zigzag training. One can witness the individuals engaging in calf exercises prior to quad exercises, and bicep exercises before focusing on the muscles of the back. Indeed, it should be noted that the back musculature possesses greater size and mass compared to the biceps, thereby necessitating the prioritization of back muscle training before focusing on the biceps. Furthermore, engaging in lighter physical activities prior to more strenuous exercises is an incorrect approach to fitness. Based on Arnold's approach to fitness and the practices of other renowned bodybuilders, it is recommended to prioritize heavier movements over lighter movements during a training session. For instance, it is advisable to perform deadlifts before lat pull downs, squats before lunges, and bench press before flyes.

Begin by incorporating foundational exercises into your fitness routine

Cables, machines, and isolation exercises do not necessitate sufficient body equilibrium, as these activities typically demand minimal to no body balance. Conversely, the exercises of back rows, overhead press, deadlifts, and squats should take precedence, given that they necessitate more precise technique and body equilibrium in order to execute them accurately.

compete your yesterday

Strive to perform optimally during your subsequent day of training in order to surpass your previous session. This implies that it is necessary for you to exhibit a higher level of intensity and enthusiasm in your performance, surpassing the standards you set for yourself yesterday. This method offers the most efficient means of achieving substantial progress within a condensed timeframe, in contrast to more protracted timelines. It represents a confidential approach employed by noteworthy bodybuilding figures from yesteryears.

Place greater emphasis on engaging in exercises that require a higher level of technical expertise

By examining renowned and accomplished Olympic champions in bodybuilding, one can discover the clandestine methods they employ to develop exceptionally muscular physiques reminiscent of iconic superheroes such as Batman and Superman. I have elaborated upon several paramount factors in cultivating increased muscle mass while concurrently attaining a more slender physique. Engaging in advanced technical exercises, which demand enhanced coordination, power, timing, speed, and technique, prior to simpler exercises, serves as a convenient method for sustaining optimal energy levels throughout your training session.

Be creative

Upon attaining an adequate understanding of bodybuilding exercises, one has the opportunity to make minor modifications to the angle of their exercises, thereby enhancing the tension and stretching effect on their muscles. One can augment muscular tension by altering their grip and foot positioning.

Alternate combinations

Your bodybuilding endeavors are being facilitated by the efficacy of your exercise regimen. Therefore, it is essential to consistently replace these tires in order to navigate this career path with utmost security. I suggest modifying your exercise regimen by making slight adjustments to the combination of routines. Incorporating a combination of flat bench and incline bench press, as well as incline bench press and parallel bar dips, would be a beneficial modification to your exercise regimen.

It is imperative not to disregard one's areas of weakness.

Most contemporary bodybuilders tend to construct their training regimen based on their areas of strength while almost disregarding their areas of weakness. Allocating focus to address one's areas of weakness can be challenging, yet it yields positive results. Renowned bodybuilders consistently place emphasis on addressing their areas of weakness in order to effectively combat their limitations and enhance their performance.

The plan should adequately account for the prevailing demands.

It is imperative to adjust and refine your training regimen as you advance in order to sustain motivation. It is advised against employing the identical strategy that was utilized during your initial stages of learning. Your exercise regimen must cater to your current needs within the ongoing process of bodybuilding.

Self-disobedience

Please exercise discipline and refrain from succumbing to the temptation of ceasing your training for the day. Stay resolute in your determination, thus inspiring others to adhere diligently to your meticulously devised regimen. The practice of self-discipline is integral to achieving success since there are instances when one's own desires may lead them astray from making prudent choices.

The perfect male body

The ideal male physique will encompass impeccably sculpted muscles. All elements will maintain their appropriate ratios.

There exists a prevalent misconception commonly referred to as body sculpting. Its primary purpose is to encourage customers to make purchases of products such as supplements, exercise training programs, and magazines.

The concept entails incorporating a multitude of exercises featuring numerous repetitions, utilizing lightweight equipment.

These methods are not at all relevant to the attainment of an ideal physique. A wide array of exercises is not necessary. There is no necessitation for extended aerobic sessions. There is no necessity for you to allocate extensive periods of time at the gym. There is no requirement for you to engage in weightlifting on a daily basis. Indeed, your utilization of the gym will be limited to three days per week.

If you adhere to this established blueprint of rationale, you can anticipate remarkable outcomes within approximately a twelve-week timeframe.

There is an abundant array of diverse body-building routines circulating. They do work. Nevertheless, their efficacy is predominantly observed among individuals who employ anabolic substances. In the case of regular fitness enthusiasts, such practices will merely result in excessive training. Consequently, negligible or no substantial development will be discernible.

An additional erroneous belief pertains to extended durations of aerobic exercise. Currently, a plethora of studies have emerged demonstrating that this specific form of training results in the depletion of muscle mass and crucial bodily tissues.

Fortunately, there has perpetually existed an exercise regime that yields positive results. You\\\'ll learn it here.

What does work

Sufficient level of intensity that exhibits a progressive augmentation.

Perfect form

The right exercises

Eating enough

Fast metabolism

Sufficient level of magnitude that continues to raise

The muscles experience an increase in size when they are exposed to heightened levels of stress. The muscles undergo adaptations in response to the increased workload.

Perfect form

Attaining optimal form is essential for achieving an ideal physique. A considerable number of individuals in fitness facilities are engaging in improper weightlifting techniques. The consequence is the development of muscular imbalance, ultimately leading to injury.

When employing appropriate technique, muscles undergo complete development and attain their optimal form.

The right exercises

There exists a multitude of exercises in the vicinity. The majority of them yield only marginal outcomes. You don\\\'t need them. Indeed, a minimal quantity is sufficient to achieve optimal physical fitness.

Eating enough

The growth of muscles is contingent upon the provision of nourishment. The adequacy of your training does not hold significance. Failure to provide sufficient nourishment to your muscles will impede their growth. Indeed, they will diminish in size.

Fast metabolism

Extended duration of aerobic exercises does not yield optimal results. In addition, they incinerate muscular tissue. There exists a significantly more straightforward and considerably more efficient approach.

Summary

Developing your musculature does not necessarily require an extensive repertoire of exercises. These routines will excessively fatigue and strain your body, leading to overtraining. They are unlikely to yield significant outcomes.

Extended periods of aerobic exercise are unnecessary. They solely incinerate muscular and tissue matter.

There is no necessity for extensive periods of time spent at the fitness center. A frequency of only thrice weekly suffices.

The four essential requirements encompass intensity, form, suitable exercises, and an adequate dietary intake.

Standing triceps press

This exercise effectively targets the entirety of the triceps region.

Please ensure that you utilize the complete extent of motion. One should experience a thorough extension at the lowermost point of the exercise.

Commence by positioning the weight in an elevated position overhead. Once more, ensconce your hands firmly around the bar to ensure secure hold and prevent slippage.

Gradually lower the weight towards the back of your head as you flex your arms. Strive to maintain a stable and upward direction of your upper arms throughout the entirety of the exercise.

Maintain a forward gaze while executing your repetitions. Looking upwards may pose a potential hazard to the occipital region of the neck, potentially resulting in injury.

Session one has concluded. During this session, the primary focus has been on exercising the chest, shoulders, and triceps muscle groups.

Session two

In this session, only two exercises focusing on the back are required. This is because these exercises effectively target and engage the comprehensive range of muscles in the back region.

The lumbar region would have already undergone significant exertion through exercises such as squats and deadlifts.

These exercises are featured in session number three.

Chin-ups wide grip

Find a chin-up bar. These can be found in nearly every fitness facility.

This exercise specifically focuses on the latissimus dorsi muscles. These are the garments that provide you with the desired tapered appearance.

Upon commencing this exercise, you can anticipate discovering it to be exceedingly challenging. Please engage in as many iterations as possible. You will improve.

If you are unable to complete a single repetition, consider utilizing a supportive surface to rest your feet upon as an aid. Utilize a durable chair or container. As your physical strength improves, you may discontinue the use of this.

If it is your desire, you have the option to affix additional mass to your physique. Nevertheless, you will discover that your body mass is adequately sufficient.

Please adhere to a maximum of six repetitions per set. Continue performing repetitions until you reach the point where executing six repetitions with impeccable form becomes difficult for you.

To establish an appropriate grip on the bar, elevate your arms and flex them at a 90-degree angle. The proper stance entails aligning your upper arms parallel to your shoulders, while pointing your forearms in an upward direction. The width of your hands has currently reached the optimal width required for this particular exercise. Please hold onto the handle at this specific width. This is precisely suitable for engaging the entire latissimus dorsi muscles.

Initiate each repetition by retracting your shoulders downward. By undertaking this activity, you will effectively activate your back muscles. It will ensure that your back is effectively engaged in the task. Alternatively, if not, your arms will bear an excessive burden of the effort.

Once more, akin to all physical activities, ensure a comprehensive execution encompassing the entirety of the motion. At the nadir of the motion, it is imperative that your shoulders achieve complete extension. When reaching the peak of the movement, endeavor to make contact between the bar and the upper region of your chest. It is inconsequential if you do not succeed. By striving to make contact with the chest, one can ensure that they are reaching the maximum height possible.

By incorporating the complete range of motion, you will guarantee the engagement of the entire muscle group.

Chin-ups reverse close-grip

This exercise places greater emphasis on the biceps muscle group and effectively targets the central region of the back.

Commence by grasping the bar with your hands positioned at a width equivalent to the width of your shoulders. Use an underhand grip. That is to say, when you grasp the bar, ensure that your palms are oriented towards the rear.

In a similar manner to the wide-grip chin-up, initiate the motion by exerting a backward and downward force using the shoulders. This will ensure effective engagement of your posterior muscles.

Once more, strive to achieve the complete extent of motion. Extend your body completely downward and elevate yourself to the maximum extent possible.

Barbell curl

This exercise will effectively engage and target the entire length of the biceps.

Commence by placing the barbell on the floor, directly in front of your position.

Grasp the bar using an under-handed grip, with your hands positioned shoulder-width apart. Envelop the thumbs securely around the bar to prevent any risk of slipping.

Elevate yourself to a standing position so that the bar is positioned in front of your upper thighs.

Ensure that the bar is fully extended towards the shoulders in a fluid, sweeping motion. Ensure that the upper arms remain stationary and in close proximity to your body throughout the entirety of the exercise. Please refrain from utilizing your arms or swaying your body to elevate the bar in an upward motion. The sole permitted motion should encompass the lower extremities of the arms.

Ensure that the arms are extended in a downward position at the bottom, and fully flexed at the top, effectively utilizing the complete range of motion.

During this session, you have engaged in exercises targeting your dorsal muscles, deltoids, and brachialis.

English-Inspired Bacon And Egg Toasted Muffin Option

Ingredients

1 large banana
¼ cup natural yogurt
1 tbsp. honey
3 slices lean non-streaky bacon (cut any excess fat off)
2 large eggs
1 wholegrain English muffin
1 tbsp. low fat butter
1 tbsp. ketchup

Preparation Method

Initially, make certain that any superfluous fat has been removed from the bacon. Place a medium-sized frying pan onto a stove set at a low-medium heat for a duration of 2 minutes. Proceed to add the oil spray and the bacon into the pan. Cook the bacon for a period of

10 minutes, ensuring to turn it frequently. Subsequently, place two eggs into a pan and pour boiling water to sufficiently cover them, then proceed to cook for a duration of 7 minutes. After the eggs are prepared, submerge them in cold water for a duration of one minute. Proceed by draining the water and delicately tapping the eggs in multiple areas using a spoon. Allow a time span of two minutes for the eggs to rest before proceeding with the peeling process. Whilst the main course simmers, take this opportunity to craft a delectable finale. Begin by finely chopping one generous-sized banana and placing it in a separate dish. Next, artfully drizzle a dollop of yogurt and a touch of honey over the banana, creating an exquisite dessert. Ultimately, once the eggs and bacon have been fully cooked, proceed to slice the muffin in half and proceed toasting it until it achieves a desired

golden brown hue. Apply the butter evenly across the surface of both halves of the bread and proceed to layer the bacon, eggs, and red sauce in between them.

Foundational Nutritional Recommendations For Individuals Engaged In Bodybuilding

If you possess any aspirations in the realm of bodybuilding or enhancing your physical appearance, the key factor lies in the domain of nutrition.

Similar to numerous other professionals in the field, it is my assertion that a substantial portion, approximately 80%, of achieving success in bodybuilding is contingent upon one's dietary choices and intake. An impressive 80% statistically validates my claim, as I have personally witnessed the outcomes on my own transformative journey. The distinguishing factor between bodybuilders and the average individual who sporadically engages in physical exercise lies in their unwavering commitment and unwavering dedication to their nutritional regimen and dietary choices. Directing one's attention towards these matters beyond the gym will pave the path to achieving success. In the gym, you are not actively growing muscle, but rather depleting it to stimulate subsequent strengthening when nourishing your body with high-quality foods and ensuring adequate rest at home.

While nutrition holds a significant level of importance for all individuals engaged in bodybuilding, it assumes paramount significance and criticality when one identifies as a Hard Gainer. Inadequate consumption of nutrient-rich calories and deviation from your designated dietary regimen can have detrimental effects on your muscular growth. Do you have any desire for that at this moment?

Guidelines for Growth:

The recommended daily protein consumption equals 1.5 grams per pound of body weight (i.e.) According to nutritional guidelines, a bodybuilder weighing 100 pounds would require a daily protein intake of 150 grams in order to support muscular development.

The recommended daily carbohydrate intake is 3 grams per pound of body weight, for instance. A bodybuilder weighing 100 pounds would require a daily intake of 300 grams of carbohydrates to facilitate muscle growth.

According to recommended guidelines, the daily consumption of 0.5 grams of fat per pound of body weight, for instance... A bodybuilder weighing 100 pounds would require an intake of 50 grams of fat per day in order to promote muscle growth.

These quantities should be gradually increased over a duration of 14 days. In order to acquire this significant amount of calories, individuals who find it challenging to gain weight should consume 6-7 evenly distributed meals on a daily basis. This implies the consumption of more frequent, smaller-sized meals with an interval of approximately 2-3 hours. This approach will guarantee the ideal assimilation of nutrients, as well as a consistent provision of nourishment to promote muscle repair and rebuilding.

As previously stated, it is recommended that your total calorie consumption be divided into 6-7 smaller portioned meals, to be consumed every 2-3 hours. If you are dedicated to the pursuit of bodybuilding and aiming to gain substantial muscle mass, the conventional practice of consuming just three meals a day consisting of breakfast, lunch, and dinner has become outdated. Regular feeding throughout the day is essential because it ensures a continuous supply of nutrients to support muscle function, while preventing the body from entering a catabolic state, a condition where the body breaks down its own muscle for energy.

Undertaking the task of preparing 6-7 nutritious meals each day can be quite challenging. Hence, it is possible to employ protein shakes and weight gainer shakes as liquid substitutes for meals. Outlined below are specific particulars regarding a typical workout day that consists of 7 meals.

Meal #1-Breakfast: 8:00am

Protein Shake

Carbohydrate source

Meal #2-Snack: 10:00am

Protein source

Carbohydrate source

Fat source

Meal #3-Lunch: 1:00pm

Protein source

Carbohydrate source

Fat source

Meal #4-Snack: 4:00pm

Protein source

Carbohydrate source

Fat source

Workout: 5:00pm

Meal #5-Post-Workout: 6:00pm

Protein Shake

Carbohydrate source

Meal #6-Dinner: 8:00pm

Protein source

Carbohydrate source

Fat source

Evening Snack before Bed: 11:00pm.

Protein beverage (for individuals weighing over 200 pounds)

Protein source

Strategies and Techniques for Slim Individuals aiming to Build Sizeable Muscle at an Accelerated Rate

If you inquire with the majority of bodybuilders, they will commonly convey that the process of training is comparatively effortless. Engaging in the demanding task of lifting massive weights and continuously pushing your body to its utmost capabilities day after day is undoubtedly an arduous endeavor. Comprehending the intricacies of bench pressing, squatting, curling, and similar exercises is not excessively challenging to acquire, particularly when one is eager to enhance their performance.

Conversely, the realm of nutrition can be intricate when it comes to determining which specific types of carbohydrates and proteins are optimal for consumption. Which vitamins and minerals are of utmost importance? In addition, bodybuilders must also keep track of aspects such as meal timing, creatine intake, and the complete range of supplements.

It can prove to be a daunting experience for individuals harboring a simple desire to engage in weightlifting and muscle development. Should you have any inquiries, it is highly probable that the answers can be found within this resource. I have meticulously gathered the most essential strategies and techniques to assist you in navigating the complex terrain of all matters pertaining to food and dietary supplements. This comprehensive overview provides a set of basic to advanced principles that have been rigorously tested and proven to be accurate and efficient.

Whether your goal is to increase muscle mass, achieve a lean physique, or maintain your current weight, you will discover invaluable information and guidance right at your disposal.

Enhancing The Dietary And Fitness Routine For The Purpose Of Developing Substantial Muscle Mass

Strength training is a vital component of any effective exercise regimen, particularly for individuals engaged in bodybuilding endeavors with the objective of enhancing muscle mass. The process of building muscle mass necessitates substantial commitment and discipline, encompassing adherence to a rigorous dietary protocol and the implementation of a tailored exercise regimen that surpasses the intensity level of a typical fitness plan. Whether your goal is to attain muscularity for its aesthetic allure or to participate in bodybuilding competitions, attaining the desired muscle mass is possible through adherence to a thoughtfully designed fitness regimen comprising both strength and cardiovascular training, in combination with a disciplined dietary approach.

Outlined below are several essential steps in the process of developing muscle mass:

Diet:

Incorporating a nutritious and rigorous dietary regimen is a fundamental element in attaining the desired outcomes for muscle hypertrophy. When seeking to develop muscle, a dietary regimen is likely to incorporate a range of substantial, yet nutritious calories. Prominent dietary choices that offer advantages for individuals aspiring to build their physique encompass nutritious sources of fats (such as fish oil or flax seed), complex carbohydrates, whey protein, turkey, chicken, tuna, an assortment of vegetables, and egg whites. Seeking expert advice from a registered dietitian is expected to be extremely advantageous in developing an optimal dietary regimen.

It is highly advisable to augment protein consumption while engaging in a comprehensive bodybuilding regimen, as it confers significant advantages in facilitating the repair and upkeep of connective tissues and muscles. The whey protein shake is expected to provide assistance in this matter. You may also wish to consider the availability of supplements such as glutamine and creatine, however, it is imperative that you thoroughly investigate the supplementation regimens before commencing with them. It is imperative to maintain proper hydration levels by consuming a substantial quantity of water, ideally at a rate of one gallon per day, to adequately meet the muscles' water requirements.

Exercise:

Implement a fitness regimen that incorporates the utilization of unfixed weights. Initiating a regimen of free weight exercises may pose initial challenges, yet their potency in yielding superior outcomes for diverse muscle groups remains unequivocal. Incorporating an adequately structured exercise routine that includes appropriate free weight lifts can lead to enhanced gains by effectively engaging the core and postural muscles. An exercise regimen comprising of pull-ups, seated dips, deadlifts, bench presses, and squats is highly likely to be beneficial.

A well-designed training regimen ought to prioritize specific sets of muscles for each individual workout, while ensuring that the same muscle group is not exercised consecutively within a 48-

hour period. It is often advised to allocate a period of 48 to 72 hours before engaging in subsequent exercise targeting the same muscle groups. It is recommended to allocate a full break of one or two consecutive days per week in order to allow for muscular recuperation and recovery.

Optimal Exercise Regimen for Muscle Gain - The Five Foundational Principles of an Ideal Resistance Training Routine

There is an abundance of workouts and exercises available to facilitate the growth and development of muscle mass. However, a majority of individuals dedicate excessive amounts of time to determining which exercises they should engage in. It is highly crucial to engage in an appropriate exercise routine. This is a pivotal factor that contributes to why certain individuals manage to achieve remarkable results after spending three hours at the gym, while others attend the gym six or even seven days a week with minimal observable outcomes. It is evident that individuals who devote a mere three hours per week to physical exercise also adhere to an outstanding dietary regimen.

1) Muscular threshold and its limits.

Muscle threshold refers to the level of physical exertion that the body is able to sustain within a defined period. Muscle development can only occur when they are stimulated accordingly. In order to enhance your muscular development, it is imperative to progressively augment the level of muscle resistance during each and every workout session.

2) Engage a maximum number of muscle fibers.

The subsequent recommendation for increasing muscle mass is to ensure that you have effectively engaged each individual muscle fiber within the specific region of the trained muscle. Every individual muscle fiber must receive training and exercise without exceptions.

To provide clarification, it is not advisable to engage in light training for a few pounds.

3) Engage in resistance training using significant load for a substantial number of repetitions.

The volume of work exerted on the muscular system exhibits a direct correlation with its potential for muscle growth and strengthening. Strive to increase productivity within the same or reduced time frame.

4) Inducing failure through training.

To elevate your muscle-building workout to a higher level, it is crucial to train until you have attained the point of muscular fatigue. Do not cease your muscular training regimen unless you have reached a point where continued movement of the weight is no longer possible.

The deliberate pursuit of failure is crucial as it guarantees the maximal utilization of muscle fibers. This is certainly one aspect that sets the three-hour-per-week individuals apart from the rest. The individuals who are excessively dedicating their time at the gym are neglecting valuable muscle fibers, thus failing to utilize and exercise them effectively.

5) Assess the level of your exertion

Rest assured that implementing these suggestions will undoubtedly yield impressive outcomes. Nonetheless, it is crucial that your intense physical exertion fosters an anabolic milieu. Maintain diligent documentation of your progress in a training journal.

If one is committed to their muscle training regimen and overall fitness, it is advisable to keep a journal. It is crucial to establish objectives for every workout session. As your level of training increases, the importance of this becomes increasingly significant.

7 Intense Workout Routines to Demonstrate Effective Methods for Building Considerable Upper Arm Power

Do you wish to acquire substantial strength in your biceps? The key is to employ innovative thinking. The subsequent 7 exercises encompass distinctive explosive bicep workouts that are not commonly practiced or may be unfamiliar to you.

Exercise 1: Single dumbbell preacher curl using a double-handed hammer grip.

Three sets with eight to twelve repetitions per set

Exercise 2: Isometric Pectoral Muscles & Bilateral Single Dumbbell Preacher Curl

Three sets with eight to twelve repetitions per set.

Exercise 3: Unilateral Towel Cable Twist Curl

Three sets with eight to twelve repetitions per set

Task 4: Perform Towel-Assisted Chin-ups

Three Sets until Failure" or "Three Sets leading to Failure" or "Three Sets until the point of Failure

Exercise Five: Towel Barbell Curls

Complete three sets with a range of eight to ten repetitions.

Exercise 6: Reverse Barbell Curls" can be restated in a formal tone as: "Task 6: Performing Reverse Barbell Curls

Three sets with eight to twelve repetitions per set

Exercise 7: Free Weight Bicep Curls using the Pinch Grip

Performing three sets with eight to twelve repetitions per set.

These exercises primarily emphasize the development of the biceps. However, incorporating the use of a towel during these exercises provides an opportunity to enhance one's grip strength. Enhancing your grasp proficiency is essential should you desire to elevate greater loads in the future and forms the foundation for attaining increased muscular strength in your biceps.

Additionally, it is of equal significance to develop further muscular strength in your forearms. Reverse barbell curls elicit significant activation in the forearms and constitute yet another pivotal exercise in augmenting bicep strength.

Engage in this exercise regimen on two occasions within a seven-day period. Initiate your initial bicep workout as a strength-focused session, ensuring to incorporate designated rest periods of 60 to 90 seconds between sets. Designate your second biceps workout of the week as a focused session on muscular endurance and conditioning. Perform the 7 exercises in a circuit format and attempt to minimize the rest periods between sets. The objective is to successfully finish a circuit without any interruptions. After concluding the circuit, it is advisable to take a brief intermission of 2 to 3 minutes before commencing again. Please perform three circuits in order to complete the workout.

As apparent, we are extensively incorporating unorthodox explosive exercises that deviate from the customary practices. The practice of employing variety in order to maintain freshness and novelty is crucial for sustaining interest in muscle training. This, in turn, plays a paramount role in promoting continuous muscle development, particularly when seeking to achieve notable strength gains in the biceps.

Chapter 2: The Do-nots

Certainly, in the realm of optimizing muscular mass development, it is imperative to not only identify a comprehensive list of recommended foods to consume in appropriate quantities, but also to recognize specific dietary items that should be avoided altogether to achieve ultimate efficacy in one's training routine. These foods, while deemed acceptable in alternative settings, can engender a deceitful perception of sustenance for individuals engaged in bodybuilding. While it is permissible to consume these food items in limited quantities, it is imperative to seek out superior alternatives whenever feasible.

Low-calorie vegetables. Indeed, it is accurate to state that vegetables offer a nourishing impact in terms of promoting overall physical fitness and well-being. The issue at hand is that a significant number of novice bodybuilders fail to consume an adequate amount of nourishment. What is the reason behind our instruction to refrain from their company? The reason behind this phenomenon lies in the fact that specific vegetables like celery and lettuce have the capacity to satiate one's appetite without simultaneously supplying an adequate amount of calories. Thus, you sense a sense of satiety despite your muscles exhibiting an ongoing demand for additional nourishment. More favorable alternatives would include produce of superior quality, such as squash and broccoli.

Simple carbohydrates. While others may strive for slender figures, bodybuilders place significant emphasis on the nutritional significance of carbohydrates, albeit of the appropriate variety. It is imperative to steer clear of sugary, processed carbohydrates at any expense. These uncomplicated carbohydrates, frequently encountered in vending machine edibles, confections, confectioneries, and refined bread, have the potential to induce fluctuating energy levels that are challenging to regulate. On the other hand, unprocessed carbohydrates like the ones present in whole-grain bread are metabolized at a slower rate, thereby sustaining energy levels for a longer duration.

Soy products. Soy has become increasingly popular as a nutritious food option and a viable substitute for meat among individuals following a vegetarian dietary pattern. Nevertheless, if you are an individual dedicated to bodybuilding, it would be wise to refrain from this alternative. The protein present in soy, despite its prevalence, exerts a comparatively lesser influence on muscle protein synthesis compared to animal-derived proteins. Furthermore, the protein present in soy is inherently deficient as it lacks certain essential amino acids typically found in meat, dairy, or fish. Hence, in order to fulfill the necessary amino acid requirements, it is imperative to combine soy protein with other protein sources.

4. Processed meat. There are numerous justifications for avoiding processed meats, and individuals who prioritize their well-being should be capable of enumerating a plethora of such reasons. Nevertheless, there exists an additional rationale for individuals engaged in muscle building to refrain from consumption of processed products. Natural meats, being rich in protein, serve as essential components for promoting muscle development. In contrast, processed meats exhibit reduced levels of overall nutrition, along with an elevation of undesirable elements detrimental to one's physiological well-being. This would entail reducing consumption of bacon,

pastrami, and baloney in favor of higher-quality, fresh meat options.

Chapter 3 - Enhancing the Limbs

You are already acquainted with the dietary regimen. This is now your opportunity to achieve parity with the masters of physical strength.

It should be noted, nonetheless, that a significant level of commitment is required for a workout to yield desired results. There is no involvement of quantum physics in this scenario. To achieve the flawlessly desirable physique you have long yearned for, a fervent dedication akin to religious fervor is essential. It is imperative to take the following actions as well:

Monitoring your progress via a dedicated personal training diary. This journal shall chronicle your initial progress, encompassing the weights and exercise regimens with which you commenced, while highlighting the subsequent enhancements achieved throughout your remarkable pursuit of physical fitness.

Continuing with each individual exercise until reaching the point of muscular fatigue or exhaustion. Failure in this context does not imply any detrimental implications; rather, it signifies that you have exerted your physical strength to the extent where it becomes unfeasible to execute another repetition of the precise exercise in question.

Allocating a maximum of one hour for your comprehensive exercise routine, encompassing warm-up activities through to cool-down exercises.

Allowing for a brief period of respite between sets within a prescribed exercise regimen.

Maintaining proper posture during the exercises. An illustrative instance would be the universally acknowledged fact that proper execution of pushups entails adhering to a correct technique, whereas an incorrect approach may lead to suboptimal results or potential injury. In any endeavor of significance, it is imperative to consistently pursue the appropriate course of action.

During periods of rest from physical exercise, it is highly advisable to prioritize ample relaxation, particularly through obtaining adequate sleep, while endeavors should be made to refrain from experiencing excessive stress.

Numerous bodybuilders departed the fitness center experiencing either physical discomfort or acute mortification, resulting from their engagement in strenuous weightlifting exercises without adhering to appropriate respiratory methods. Inquire with your fitness instructor regarding the appropriate methods of respiration in order to avoid any inadvertent mishaps when utilizing the barbell equipment.

Ensuring observance of nutritional and supplemental requirements.

In this chapter, we commence with exercises designed to strengthen the body's extremities. The extremities, namely the arms and legs, are likely the most prominently visible areas of the attired human physique and hold significant significance for individuals following a regimen focused on physical fitness and muscular development. There is no need to explicitly declare your fitness endeavors to others, as the well-toned muscles on your arms and legs will silently but effectively demonstrate the efforts you have put into your physical training.

The appendages - On numerous occasions in the past, have you encountered celestial beings donned in well-fitted garments, wherein the sleeves can scarcely confine an abundance of exquisitely chiseled musculature? Acknowledge it - it is undeniable that your gaze fixated on those formidable and aesthetically pleasing biceps, or perhaps you yearn to possess robust arm muscles of your own.

There are numerous exercises and regimens accessible for the purpose of developing well-defined arm muscles.

Biceps. At present, the practice of performing bicep curls using light weights stands out as the prevailing exercise method for effectively sculpting and strengthening the biceps. In order to perform the correct bicep curl, it is necessary to adhere to the subsequent guidelines:

(1) Begin by extending the arm downward along the anterior portion of the corresponding thigh, with the hand holding the weight.

(2) Execute a flexion of the elbow in an arc-like motion, directed towards the shoulder on the corresponding side, while holding the weight.

(3) Contract the muscle as the dumbbell reaches the shoulder.

(4) Lower the weight gradually until it reaches the level of the thigh.

(5) Perform the sequence of actions on ten occasions, dividing them into three distinct groups or sets.

Naturally, subsequent to completing the procedure with one arm, proceed to replicate the exact same process with the other arm. Exercise caution when regulating the motion of the arm, particularly during its descent towards the thigh. These curls can be performed either unilaterally, beginning with one arm followed by the other, or sequentially, in one series.

Triceps and brachialis. Frequently, the triceps are commonly overlooked in favor of the biceps, primarily owing to the appealing nature attributed to the latter. Nevertheless, it is important to note that the triceps account for approximately two-thirds of the overall musculature of the upper arm. Consequently, it is imperative that equal emphasis is placed on the development and care of these particular muscle groups.

Conversely, the brachialis muscle is situated directly beneath the biceps. When the arm is flexed through the bending of the elbow joint, the circular muscular region visible on the lateral aspect of the upper arm is known as the brachialis. Both the biceps and triceps muscles necessitate a comprehensive exercise routine to achieve aesthetically pleasing arms.

Utilizing dumbbells, an effective exercise for enhancing the triceps and brachialis is the single-arm overhead tricep extension. Prior to engaging in this exercise, it is imperative to ensure that your body assumes a perpendicular posture, be it in a standing or seated position. The following procedure is to be adhered to:

(1) Elevate the arm carrying the weight to a position located prominently above the head.

(2) Gradually lower the weight towards the lower part of the neck in a deliberate manner, ensuring that the upper arm is fixed at a 90-degree angle with respect to the rest of the body.

(3) Elevate the arm to its original position.

(4) Execute the procedure on ten occasions, divided among three sets.

It is imperative that one maintains control and executes proper form while carrying out this routine, as failure to do so may result in potential injury to the neck and/or head.

A cable pulley can serve as an effective alternative to dumbbells in performing the triceps/brachialis exercise, as the cables can be manipulated using a comparable technique to that used with weights.

The lower extremities - We have observed numerous bodybuilders exhibiting well-developed upper limbs, prominent chests, impressive abdominal muscles, and broad shoulders -- juxtaposed with disproportionately underdeveloped lower limbs. We aim to avoid finding ourselves in this predicament; therefore, we have implemented a procedure to assist you in developing muscularity in the legs.

Prior to proceeding, it is essential to acknowledge that in the majority of these exercises, there will be a absence of intermission or reprieve between each set. Furthermore, the frequency ranges between 10 and 15 sets, constituting approximately 30 to 45 minutes of your overall workout. It is advisable to incorporate the use of weights when engaging in the aforementioned exercises. All of these exercises have been specifically designed to effectively target and develop the muscles in your thighs, hamstrings, and calves, which are essential for achieving the desired strength and tone.

Lunges. Perform five sets comprising of ten repetitions each, without any intervals for rest.

Leg curls. Perform five sets comprising of fifteen repetitions each, without taking any breaks. This can be achieved with or without the use of weights; nevertheless, the likelihood of developing more robust and well-defined hamstring muscles in the shortest possible timeframe is notably higher when performing leg curls with the addition of weights.

Squats. Perform five sets of ten repetitions, interspersed with one minute of rest.

Standing calf raises. Engage in a minimum of 20 repetitions per set, performing a total of six sets for this exercise, while allowing only a brief rest period of 20 to 30 seconds in between each set. The key here lies in focusing one's attention on the process by which the calf muscles undergo contraction.

Tips For Enhancing Muscular Development For All Individuals

Initiating a muscle building regimen can prove to be quite arduous for individuals lacking guidance on commencing their journey. This concise article will provide you with insights on various approaches to begin. If you are inclined to embark on a journey of muscular development, then proceed to peruse this article and commence your endeavors promptly!

If your goal is specifically to enhance muscle development rather than overall fitness improvement, it is advised to refrain from engaging in concurrent strength training and cardiovascular exercises. The justification behind this occurrence lies in the fact that these two forms of physical activity elicit contradicting physiological responses within the body. Focusing solely on muscle acquisition will enhance your results.

Ensure that you obtain sufficient rest during the nocturnal hours. It is essential to allow sufficient time for your muscles to undergo the necessary repair process following the strain imposed during a weight lifting session. Insufficient rest for the muscles can significantly diminish the effectiveness of your workout.

Creatine

Are you attempting to increase your muscle mass? If you are consuming nutritionally dense foods, engaging in intense physical exercise but have not yet achieved the desired outcomes, you may contemplate incorporating creatine supplements to enhance muscle development. Creatine facilitates the development of muscular hypertrophy, unequivocally. It is not merely favored among numerous professional bodybuilders; it is also markedly utilized by a multitude of elite athletes across various sports.

Some common sense. Please ensure that you consult a medical professional regarding any dietary supplements that you may need to refrain from consuming. You potentially have the capacity to optimize your muscle-building endeavors through the utilization of substances like creatine, protein, or alternative supplements; however, it is imperative to ascertain their respective impact on your overall well-being and soundness. The overarching principle is to ensure that no detrimental consequences arise from your endeavors to enhance muscularity through supplement usage. Undertake the task in a manner that promotes wellness.

Nitric Oxide

Utilize arginine as a means to enhance the size of your muscles. This distinct compound amplifies nitric oxide synthesis within the organism, thereby augmenting blood circulation towards the musculature. As a result, there is an increase in the transportation of hormones, oxygen, and nutrients to regions where they can have the greatest positive impact. Furthermore, this augments the levels of growth hormone. Consume a quantity of three to five grams before and directly following physical exercise. It is crucial to verify that the dose ingested after your workout is devoid of stimulants when engaging in late night exercise sessions.

Summary

Creatine supplementation should be approached cautiously, particularly when considering long-term usage. Individuals with renal conditions are strongly advised to abstain from its consumption entirely. Creatine has the potential to induce cardiac arrhythmia and muscular cramping. Adolescents who consume creatine face the most significant susceptibility. Employ creatine supplementation judiciously by adhering to the recommended safe dosage.

Incorporating an adequate amount of protein into your diet is essential for the development of muscle mass. This issue can be resolved quite conveniently through the utilization of protein shakes. They provide considerable advantages following a workout as well as prior to going to sleep. In order to expedite the process of converting fat into muscle, it

73

is advisable to consume a single protein shake on a daily basis. In the event of a different preference, it is suggested to consume 2 or 3 shakes daily to attain a desired outcome of increased weight and muscle mass.

Nitric Oxide: Employ the use of arginine to enhance muscle growth, ensuring that the post-workout dosage is devoid of stimulants. This holds particular significance during nocturnal exercise sessions.

If you are highly focused on achieving results and are seeking expedited muscle building outcomes across multiple dimensions, it would be prudent to contemplate the utilization of dietary supplements. Please ensure that you undertake the task with utmost caution and intelligence. To your improved fitness. It is hoped that you can utilize the methodologies and suggestions provided in this article to commence your transformations at the present moment.

10. Optimal Bicep Exercise Regimen - Strategies for Enhancing Bicep Size

An often-overlooked fact about biceps is that their workout holds equal importance to other exercise routines, as they play a vital role in the overall fitness of your body, particularly if you engage in gym training. However, it is important to note that the development of biceps is not an instantaneous process. It necessitates dedicated time at the gym, along with patience, consistency, and adherence to a regular workout schedule.

It is likely that you have come across numerous articles pertaining to techniques for increasing bicep size, as well as the most effective workouts for developing the biceps. build muscles fast ? tips for biceps size? However, it is important to note that merely attempting these exercises without proper guidance may yield limited or no results. Therefore, I implore you not to lose hope. By carefully absorbing the contents of this article, you will acquire invaluable knowledge on the most effective bicep workout routines capable of sculpting your desired biceps.

Bicep Workout Routines
1. The standing barbell curl is regarded as the foremost and highly impactful exercise for enhancing bicep size. It serves as a vital workout that endows strength to the biceps, resulting in robust development. By executing this exercise correctly, visible and significant advancements in bicep size can be observed within a month.

Advice – It is important to avoid displaying arrogance while at the gym, as ego can be detrimental to your progress. Remember, you are engaging in your training for your own personal growth, rather than for the validation of others. Therefore, it is advisable to consistently challenge yourself with weights that are appropriate for your abilities, instead of attempting to lift excessively heavy weights.

2. Ez bar curl – This particular exercise holds significant importance and is often disregarded by trainees during their bicep workouts. It not only aids in achieving bicep mass, but also enhances bicep definition and peak. The Ez bar curl is executed with an Ez bar, also referred to as a zig zag bar.

Recommendation: It is highly advised to always incorporate Ez bar curl exercises into your training regimen. This particular exercise has been proven to effectively expedite the growth of your biceps in comparison to other bicep workouts.

3. Preacher curl - The preacher curl exercise entails sitting on a preacher bench and utilizing an EZ bar. Alternatively, if your gym is equipped with an adjustable preacher machine, you may also perform this exercise. Regarded as an exceptional bicep workout, the prominent figure Arnold has acclaimed its effectiveness in shaping and developing the bicep peak.

Recommendation: It is advised to refrain from using a straight barbell during preacher curl workouts, and instead opt for an ez barbell. Always ensure to prioritize three key aspects when engaging in any exercise routine: proper form, controlled speed, and suitable weight.

4. Concentration curls are a highly effective exercise targeting the biceps muscles, resulting in an increase in size and mass. This exercise involves the use of dumbbells while seated on a bench and can be categorized as a high-intensity workout.

Recommendations - In the case of being an advanced trainee, standing Concentration curls may be performed. It is advisable to refrain from utilizing dumbbells of excessive weight.

5. The hammer curl exercise is effective in shaping and toning the biceps, while also enhancing forearm strength. One may opt to use either a dumbbell or a rope for this exercise, but it is recommended to primarily utilize a dumbbell in order to maximize bicep strengthening benefits.

Recommendation: It is advised to utilize a moderate weight while performing the hammer curl exercise in order to achieve immediate noticeable effects on the biceps. Additionally, incorporating a higher number of repetitions per set, ideally aiming for a minimum of 15, will facilitate the development of both the desired shape and size.

Consequently, the highly effective session of bicep exercise has concluded. Commence your fitness regimen from this day forth, as you bear sole responsibility for shaping your own fate.

Muscle Overview

In terms of enhancing physical fitness and aesthetics, mere weight loss proves insufficient. Increasing muscle mass is, in fact, the key to maintaining a slender physique and plays a pivotal role in enhancing overall physical strength.

While possessing substantial muscular mass might contribute to an increase in one's weight as indicated by a scale, this should not be a cause for concern. Having a well-developed musculature would not contribute to the perception of being overweight, but rather impart a sense of being sculpted and exceptionally robust. Even during ordinary tasks such as carrying weighty bags of groceries or commuting to work, your charm remains ever present.

"Below are additional justifications for why the augmentation of muscle mass is imperative:

Engaging in physical activity without incorporating weight-bearing exercises and strength training may render you more prone to sustaining injuries. The sole means to prevent physical degeneration in one's body is by enhancing bone density, a feat that can solely be achieved through the development of muscle mass. Engaging in a consistent routine of lifting heavy weights results in the strengthening of the body's connective tissues, thereby leading to a subsequent enhancement in bone density.

The presence of well-developed musculature contributes to enhanced sleep patterns, regulation of blood sugar levels, enhanced mental well-being, as well as improved balance and stability.

The augmentation of muscle mass accordingly heightens your metabolic rate. With an accelerated metabolism, it becomes attainable to effectively burn calories during periods of rest. According to experts, one pound of muscle has the capacity to expend 6 calories per day. Consider the potential caloric expenditure even without engaging in physical activity!

As a consequence of the post-exercise oxygen consumption phenomenon, your body will experience a doubled calorie burn following your weight training session. Doesn't it render the agony entirely justifiable?

With well-developed musculature, the performance of daily tasks will be executed with minimal strain and exertion. Ascending multiple levels of stairs, tending to the lawn with a lawnmower, and heaving cumbersome furniture will no longer be perceived as arduous tasks.

The musculature of the human anatomy is intricate and captivating. In addition to enhancing your physical appearance and enabling you to handle weighty objects, it is imperative to understand that your muscular system serves additional purposes.

Understanding Muscles

Every person possesses more than 700 muscles within their body. These muscles comprise resilient tissues, analogous to a rubber band, and contain tens of thousands of fibers. Muscular tissue is distributed throughout the entire human body, extending beyond the biceps region.

Similar to the cardiac and cerebral organs, muscles assume critical functions within the human body. They serve as the prime motivators for your physical entity, enabling you to propel and mobilize yourself. In the absence of muscular strength, one would find it impossible to engage in any form of locomotion, from even the simplest act of moving one's lips to articulate speech, to the seemingly effortless action of fluttering one's eyelids.

Muscles Types

Your musculature is classified into three distinct types. These structures include the smooth muscle, the skeletal muscle, and the cardiac muscle.

Smooth muscles, otherwise referred to as visceral muscles, are situated within various anatomical structures such as blood vessels, stomach, intestines, bladder, and the female reproductive system including the uterus. Renowned for their involuntary nature, smooth muscles are not subject to direct control by the conscious mind. They consistently carry out their duties without causing you any concern.

Smooth muscles possess the ability to undergo elongation while sustaining a uniform level of tension over extended durations. For instance, your bladder muscles undergo relaxation to enable urine retention, subsequently inducing contraction to facilitate the expulsion of urine at the appropriate timing.

Cardiac muscles, which are a type of involuntary muscle, exclusively reside within the confines of the heart. The primary role of these muscles is to circulate blood throughout the entirety of the body. The structure of the cardiac muscles is characterized by remarkable strength, allowing them to endure the task of pumping blood continuously over the course of an individual's lifetime without experiencing strain. It additionally exhibits resistance against hypertension.

Skeletal muscles, in stark contrast to smooth muscles, are commonly recognized as the exclusive voluntary muscles of the human body. This indicates that voluntary control can be exerted over this specific group of muscles. These muscles shall remain immobile unless you so desire. The utilization of skeletal muscles is imperative for the execution of any self-initiated bodily movements such as walking, raising a hand, or scratching one's head.

Skeletal muscles exhibit variations in their morphological characteristics. The back and neck house the largest and most robust skeletal muscles in the human body. These muscular groups facilitate an erect posture and enable the freedom of movement in the neck in various orientations.

TRAINING DAY BREAKDOWN

PREPARATION - Just like in any type of physical exercise, it is vital to properly warm up your muscles, particularly the targeted muscles, to ensure adequate blood flow. This is crucial to prevent injuries and enhance muscle performance to its fullest potential. It is crucial to prioritize enhanced circulation throughout the entire body as a prerequisite, subsequently attending to the specific muscle group(s) being engaged in the exercise.

Engaging in any type of moderate aerobic exercise will result in an elevation of your heart rate, leading to a subsequent enhancement in blood circulation throughout the body. Furthermore, it would be increasingly advantageous to engage in a cardiovascular exercise that incorporates both the upper and lower extremities. This holds particularly true when the target musculature resides within the upper body (in this instance, the legs) in order to guarantee a sufficient supply of blood to this region.

An exemplary illustration would be an elliptical or stair-climber apparatus, which effectively engages both the upper and lower muscle groups of your body, furnishing a comprehensive and impartial warm-up for your entire physique. Utilizing a treadmill or a stationary bicycle predominantly directs attention towards facilitating a warm-up routine for the lower extremities and abdominal region, which is suitable when emphasizing a workout concentrated on leg exercises. A duration of 10 to 12 minutes engaging in aerobic activity at a moderate intensity level should prove adequate.

EXTENSION - Like any other physical endeavor, engaging in stretching exercises is a vital component of your warm-up regimen. As part of the weight training session, it is necessary to begin with a few warm-up sets. These sets will primarily concentrate on stretching and warming up the leg muscles, as demonstrated in the following examples:

Commence the leg stretching exercise by inclining at the waist and placing your right hand on the edge of the bench or chair. Subsequently, elevate your left foot towards the back and secure your ankle with your left hand. Furthermore, proceed by inclining your body forward at the hip joint while providing support to your upper body using your right hand, and exert an upward force on your left ankle. Please maintain the position for a duration of 15 seconds, carefully elongating the quadriceps muscles at the front of your raised leg, while simultaneously stretching the hamstring muscles at the back of your stationary leg. Please proceed with the same steps for the leg on the opposite side. Perform this stretching exercise five repetitions for each leg.

Warm-up Sets - During the initial two sets of Workout #1, it is recommended to execute the primary superset for each exercise using a modest load, enabling you to effortlessly complete 20-25 repetitions with proper technique, prior to reaching the point of muscle failure.

For the subsequent 2 sets (Workout #1), select a weight that affords a comparable range of 15-20 repetitions. The last two sets are to be executed using the designated weight you had meticulously determined for today's training session.

Your target muscles should be adequately primed by the time you finish your first superset of Exercise Routine #1. As a result, you will be able to execute Exercise Routine #2 using the weight determined for your training session.

The load applied to your training sets should be such that it enables you to execute approximately 15 repetitions in a controlled manner, with the final repetition being significantly challenging but not reaching the point of complete muscular failure. It would be advisable to ascertain the respective weights a day in advance of your scheduled training day in order to optimize efficiency. Following a brief preliminary exercise, proceed to complete one or two sets until you have determined the appropriate weight for each exercise, subsequently documenting these weights in your training log. This will obviate any uncertainties and unproductive utilization of time during your training day.

THE WORKOUTS

The exercise movements selected for the subsequent workout routines have demonstrated optimal effectiveness and demand minimal reliance on training equipment. It is advised against substituting alternative exercise movements for the ones listed below, unless you have knee or back concerns, in which case Leg Presses or squats are suggested as suitable alternatives.

The subsequent information provides a comprehensive breakdown of the sets, repetitions, and exercise motions executed for Workout 1 and Workout 2, accompanied by fundamental visual representations for each exercise movement:

Training Frequency

The frequency of training provides an essential answer to the query regarding the ideal number of times one should engage in muscle group workouts within a given week. If due attention was devoted to the volume segment, it is likely that one is already aware that, in the majority of instances, the response should exceed a mere singular occurrence.

Certain frequency studies indicate that for the majority of individuals, it is generally advisable to engage in muscle group training sessions ranging from two to four times per week, taking into account variations in experience levels and specific muscle groups. (as exemplified by a study conducted in 2016 by Schoenfield and colleagues)

In the majority of instances, the process of post-workout muscle-protein synthesis, which pertains to the growth of muscles, is typically concluded within a span of approximately two to three days, and sometimes, it may even occur at an accelerated pace. Consequently, it is reasonable to posit that muscular growth takes place on the initial day following the workout session, and potentially on the subsequent day as well. Possibly still remaining on the third. However, what about the fourth, fifth, and sixth days?

Alternatively, allow me to rephrase the statement: What is the rationale behind waiting a full week to resume muscle training when it can already undergo growth in less than half that duration? Undoubtedly, a more effective stimulus can be generated by consolidating your weekly volume into a single session. However, one must also consider the potential consequences of an improved stimulus, as it might result in the squandering of three to four days that could otherwise be allocated towards muscular development. Furthermore, it should be noted that surpassing the threshold of approximately 10-12 sets per session may result in an inefficient allocation of time at the gym, as any further increase in volume during the same day would yield negligible benefits. This is a point worth considering for proponents of the bro-split routine.

However, this does not imply that bro-splits are ineffective or should be completely avoided. Numerous other studies have found no discernible muscle-building advantages when comparing low-frequency training splits with high-frequency training splits for hypertrophy, as long as the volume of these splits is equalized. Nevertheless, this is an important consideration as one can readily incorporate additional exercises and increase training volume when employing a high-frequency split as opposed to a low-frequency split. Nevertheless, this implies that bro-splits can be considered as a viable alternative for individuals who follow a low-volume training regimen or are novices with lower volume needs.

With that being said, I firmly believe that increasing the frequency of training is beneficial for enhancing the productivity and quality of one's volume, irrespective of their skill level, be it a novice or an intermediate. It is important to bear in mind that the efficacy of each subsequent set considerably diminishes over the course of a workout. As an illustration, incorporating ten rounds of quad-compound movements within a single workout is apt to generate a highly effective stimulus. Nevertheless, you may find yourself departing the gym on hands and knees, possibly experiencing nausea, and enduring such pronounced muscular discomfort that assuming a seated position on the toilet will prove challenging for several days. All those efforts were undertaken merely to achieve marginal improvements in performance.

If you were to perform five sets of quads on Monday and an additional five sets on Thursday, the resultant level of per-workout stimulus would be approximately reduced to 80-85%, compared to performing all sets consecutively. Nevertheless, you would obtain these 80-85% on two separate occasions each week. Furthermore, the level of exhaustion would be significantly reduced compared to completing all ten sets consecutively. It is plausible that additional quad volume can be incorporated into your training regimen, thereby potentially resulting in greater muscular development.

Allow us to consolidate all the advantages inherent in training a specific muscle group at least twice weekly as opposed to adhering to a bro-split approach:

Reduced instances of fatigue and muscle soreness after each session.

There is a capacity for an increase in the (efficient) output per week.

The efficacy of volume increases per session remains higher." "The effectiveness of volume increases per session remains augmented." "The increment in volume per session maintains greater efficacy.

Two or more weekly stimuli for growth.

Multiple opportunities for advancement

Exercises targeting the identical muscle group do not exert as significant an adverse influence on one another.

Based on the aforementioned advantages, I strongly advocate incorporating a minimum of two workout sessions per week per muscle group into your training regimen.

However, considering the potential benefits of having two sessions, it stands to reason that three sessions would be even more advantageous, and perhaps four sessions would be even more beneficial than three. Why not consider implementing a training regimen that targets all muscle groups on a daily basis and necessitates an intense, all-encompassing approach?

Initially, it is important to note that the principle of diminishing returns is equally applicable to the frequency of training. Although engaging in training a muscle group twice a week is more advantageous than training it only once, the marginal benefits of increasing the frequency to three sessions per week diminish significantly, if any exist at all. The advantages of transitioning from a three-day schedule to a four-day schedule are diminished even further. This occurrence primarily arises when one reaches a point where proper recovery between sessions becomes increasingly difficult due to the excessive volume, potentially leading to a significant decline in the quality of one's workouts. In contrast, opting for high-frequency training when adhering to a low to moderate weekly volume necessitates appropriately distributing the workload across the individual workout days. There may come a time when it is necessary to achieve a particular minimum volume per session in order to elicit a favorable response. However, it is important to note that performing only one or two sets per workout may no longer be sufficient.

Nevertheless, it should be noted that certain muscle groups may possess the ability to withstand remarkably high (or at the very least, higher) frequencies and volumes. As an illustration, it can be observed that the musculature of the forearms, abdominal region, and calves, being primarily suited for endurance-oriented activities, are likely to develop a capacity to tolerate frequent training sessions once a regular training regimen has been established. This phenomenon may also be observed in other muscle groups. For instance, throughout my tenure as a trainee, I ascertained that my biceps and chest exhibit remarkably rapid recuperation, enabling me to engage them thrice weekly without detriment to my overall recovery process. Conversely, my hamstrings have gained a reputation for remaining tender for an extended duration, hence, increasing their frequency is an infrequent occurrence for me.

Additionally, your training frequency is contingent upon your level of exertion (which we shall discuss in detail subsequently) and the extent of training within each session. By consistently avoiding reaching the point of muscle failure (which is not recommended) and performing a minimal number of sets, it is probable that you will be able to train a muscle more frequently compared to completely exhausting it during your exercise sessions.

However, I am digressing. As is evident, these programming factors are interconnected and exert mutual influence on one another. Therefore, depending on the factors you prioritize, it becomes necessary to limit or reduce the emphasis on certain other factors in order to maintain the sustainability of your training, particularly throughout a mesocycle.

Therefore, it is advisable to commence with a frequency of two weekly sessions per major muscle group, incorporating a low to moderate volume, and adjust accordingly as needed. Upon the realization that certain muscle groups exhibit rapid recovery, it is advisable to incorporate an additional day of training specifically dedicated to these muscle groups. For more comprehensive information on this subject matter, please refer to the section titled "Adding Frequency" within this book.

Chapter Summary

Training frequency refers to the frequency or rate at which an individual engages in training sessions for a specific muscle group on a weekly basis.

It is advisable to maintain a minimum frequency of training each muscle at least twice per week, distributing your overall training volume reasonably evenly across your workout sessions.

Based on the individual's capacity for muscle group recovery and the amount of training volume, it may be possible to further elevate training frequency, though it is generally recommended to keep it within four sessions per week for optimal training outcomes.

Insufficient frequency levels (such as bro-splits) may prove suitable for individuals at the novice level (who experience prolonged muscle soreness and train well below the maximum volume threshold per session). However, it is highly probable that elevated frequencies yield superior results for individuals at the intermediate stage.

Adding To Food

Currently, there is extensive discourse surrounding the topic of gastrointestinal well-being. Regarding the potential advantages of incorporating probiotics and prebiotics into your dietary regimen.

The question of greater significance is how could it possibly be of no assistance?

The culmination of various physiological processes within our bodies results in the formation of a single cohesive entity. If a single component within the unit experiences an impact, the entire unit is inevitably influenced, be it in a detrimental or favorable manner. The manner in which your stomach feels, whether content or displeased, will greatly influence the outcome of your day and physical exercise. That seems obvious.

The intestinal flora is responsible for the production of the majority of serotonin in your body. Therefore, an individual who experiences contentment is essentially a product of a nourished gastrointestinal system that harbors a thriving community of beneficial microbes.

Subsequently, it becomes imperative to incorporate both probiotics and prebiotics into your physiological system. In unison, they have a direct impact on one's athletic performance.

The integration of both has already demonstrated significant efficacy in combating various diseases and ailments. Researchers hold the belief that probiotics, in combination with the prebiotics that nurture them, may engender advantageous consequences on a broad spectrum of additional medical ailments presently undergoing investigation.

PROBIOTICS

Probiotics encompass various types of microorganisms, including live bacteria, parasites, viruses, and yeast, that occur naturally within the gastrointestinal tract. The typical human gastrointestinal system harbors a diverse array of approximately 500 to 2,000 distinct species of microorganisms.

They enhance muscular recuperation, inhibit the proliferation of detrimental bacteria within the body, and contribute to the maintenance of a robust gastrointestinal system. This is achieved by facilitating the transport of food along your intestines by influencing the neural regulation of gastrointestinal motility.

Probiotics have been historically employed in the context of fermented foods and cultured dairy products.

Numerous factors prevalent in contemporary times and routine activities detrimentally affect the inherent beneficial probiotic bacteria that reside within our physiological systems. Primary harm originates from pharmaceuticals, antibiotics, cereals, sucrose, genetically modified organisms in food, and chemically treated tap water.

There are numerous justifications for the incorporation of probiotics into your dietary regimen, and the positive impact that these supplements can potentially have on your bodybuilding endeavors appears unequivocal.

As an additional resource, it is noteworthy that the FDA has categorized probiotics as a form of sustenance, rather than a pharmaceutical product.

The following are the prevailing species:

Lactobacillus acidophilus

Lactobacillus bulgarius

Lactobacillus reuteri

Streptococcus thermophilus

Saccharomyces boulardii

Bifidobacterium bifidum

Bacillus subtilis

ACTIVE PROBIOTIC FOODS

The following is a compilation of the foods that are most frequently encountered and contain live microorganisms known as probiotics:

Dairy kefir

Coconut kefir

Sauerkraut

Buttermilk

Kimchi

Kombucha

Yogurt containing live active cultures or Greek yogurt.

Unpasteurized cheese (with goat or sheep varieties being the richest).

Apple cider vinegar containing the bacterial culture known as 'mother of vinegar'

Salted gherkin pickles

Brine-cured olives

Tempeh

Miso

Natto (fermented soybeans)

Kvass, a beverage crafted through the process of fermenting aged rye bread.

If you opt to incorporate probiotics into your dietary routine as a nutritional supplement, the manner and locale of their consumption will influence the particular format you select for their usage.

They are available in various distinct shapes. Certain specimens consist of freeze-dried microorganisms that do not necessitate refrigeration. These options offer enhanced versatility, are conveniently enclosed in capsules, and facilitate easy portability.

Certain individuals are alive and possess a sensitivity to heat, thus necessitating the maintenance of refrigerated conditions for their wellbeing. This limitation curtails their ability to move around, particularly when they are constantly on the move and not staying at their residence. The available options include both powdered and liquid forms; however, it should be noted that liquid probiotics offer the highest level of purity and freshness.

PREBIOTICS

All substances classified as prebiotics fall under the category of dietary fiber, however, it should be noted that not all fibers can be classified as prebiotics. They are indigestible carbohydrates that function as sustenance for the probiotic microorganisms within your gastrointestinal tract. Due to their indigestible nature, they undergo fermentation within the intestinal tract. Fermentation promotes the proliferation of beneficial bacteria that subsequently nourish the probiotics. It\\\'s a balanced union.

There is scientific evidence to support the notion that prebiotics facilitate the absorption of minerals by the human body. They lend support to cardiovascular well-being and cognitive processes, facilitate sleep, enhance digestion, provide protection against specific cancers, regulate blood sugar levels, and manage blood pressure. They possess inherent detoxifying properties and enhance the immunity of your body. Medical professionals assert that a significant proportion of one's immune system, specifically 70 percent, is attributed to the state of their gut health. A diverse selection of nutritious prebiotic foods is available.

Dandelion greens

Jerusalem artichoke (sunchokes)

Garlic

Onions

Leeks

Asparagus

Carrots

Radishes

Cucumbers

Beets

Cabbage

Bananas, particularly those that are slightly unripe, contain an elevated level of prebiotics.

Apples
Berries
Mango
Tomatoes
Coconut
Barley
Oats
Elephant yams
Burdock root
Yacon root
Jicama root
Chicory root
Ginger root
Pure cocoa
Raw honey
Flax seeds
Chia seeds
Hemp seeds
Pumpkin seeds
Wild rice
Wheat bran
Seaweed
Acacia gum, which is present in certain dietary supplements,

When considering the incorporation of prebiotics into one's diet, it is advisable to commence with a modest quantity due to the substantial variations in individuals' dietary intake and digestive well-being. Take into consideration your emotions and proceed accordingly. Record all the particulars in your journal.

Should you experience digestive discomfort such as gas or bloating following the consumption of a small quantity of prebiotics, it would indicate a limited tolerance to dietary fiber in your body. Proceed with caution as you embark on the journey to enhance your digestive well-being.

As you augment your fiber intake, ensure a proportional increase in your water consumption. This holds significance as water facilitates the movement of fiber within your gastrointestinal system, thereby acting as a preventive measure against constipation.

SUPPLEMENTS AND VITAMINS

There is a significant amount of discussion surrounding the necessity of implementing supplements. There is an argument put forth by certain individuals positing that if one adheres to a diet that is entirely balanced and mindful, there should be no need for any form of dietary supplementation.

For the purpose of achieving physical strength and overall fitness, it is indeed accurate to state that a well-balanced diet consisting of nutritious whole foods, supplemented by a daily intake of a multivitamin, can provide all the necessary requirements. Nevertheless, bodybuilding necessitates a greater commitment from one's physique than mere conventional fitness. In order to maximize the potential of one's physical capabilities, it is imperative to provide one's body with increased attention and care. That is when the supplementation of protein-rich powders and other dietary sources intended to bolster muscle development becomes imperative.

It is essential to ensure that your diet and dietary supplements sufficiently provide the energy required to cope with more rigorous training. Insufficient fulfillment of your nutritional requirements in relation to the energy expenditure during your workout will impede your ability to effectively recuperate. You may experience significant fatigue, encounter discomfort in your joints and muscles, and potentially witness muscular tissue degradation as it attempts to regenerate the necessary resources. This phenomenon is scientifically referred to as muscular catabolism. It\\\'s very counter-productive.

The manner in which one chooses to supplement is entirely a matter of personal preference.

As a novice, there is a significant amount of information to absorb. An array of shelves filled with numerous varieties of supplements, hormones, vitamins, antioxidants, energy enhancers, performance enhancers, metabolism accelerators, endurance products, essential oils, amino acids, meal replacements, and an abundance of attractively packaged bottles adorned with vibrant colors and images depicting muscular figures vying for your attention.

There is a multitude of options available, and based on prevailing opinions, it appears that at least half of them fail to meet expectations or yield novel outcomes.

Presented below are the foremost six products that appear to possess indispensability and garner widespread consensus for optimal performance:

Whey Protein

Whey protein is unparalleled in terms of its superior absorbability. It is beneficial to consume protein early in the morning to facilitate efficient absorption following a period of rest. It is also beneficial when consumed prior to sleeping and is commonly utilized immediately following exercise.

Creatine

Creatine enhances skeletal muscle growth and significantly augments increases in physical strength. It enhances energy levels, thereby enabling one to engage in more rigorous training. In addition, it promotes the hydration of the muscle tissues, thereby resulting in their augmentation and fortification.

Beta-Alanine

Research has demonstrated that Beta-Alanine effectively augments the capacity for sustained muscle performance. Numerous individuals assert that they are capable of executing one or two supplementary repetitions during their gym sessions when engaging in sets ranging from 8 to 15. It also enhances cardiovascular performance in activities with moderate to high intensity levels, such as rowing or sprinting.

L-Glutamine

L-Glutamine is a fundamental amino acid of utmost importance in the process of muscle recuperation. It is typically administered up to four times per day to maintain a continuous supply in the body.

"Branched-Chain Amino Acids (BCAA)" can be expressed in a more formal tone as "Amino acids with a branched-chain structure (BCAA)".

Indispensable amino acids, branched-chain amino acids (BCAAs) must be consumed alongside your meals, as they play a crucial role in promoting rapid muscle recovery and facilitating protein synthesis.

Omega-3 Fish Oil

Omega-3 fatty acids facilitate efficient blood flow, thereby enabling the delivery of essential nutrients, such as protein and carbohydrates, to the muscles. They greatly enhance your metabolic rate, fortify immunity, and offer numerous advantages in combatting illness and disease.

A primary focus on developing muscle necessitates adequate intake of a subset of 12 pivotal vitamins, minerals, and nutrients. It is imperative to ensure the comprehensive incorporation of all of them in your dietary and supplementation strategies.

Calcium plays a pivotal role in the prevention of diseases and contributes to the overall well-being of the bones, heart, muscles, and nerves.

Biotin supports various physiological processes including metabolism, blood glucose regulation, hair and skin health, nail strength, brain function, cardiovascular well-being, as well as thyroid and adrenal gland functionality.

Riboflavin, also known as Vitamin B12, plays a crucial role in the process of energy production.

Iron plays a crucial role in various physiological processes, such as blood hemoglobin production, muscle function regulation, brain function maintenance, and body temperature regulation.

Copper plays a pivotal role in various biological processes such as the synthesis of melanin, maintaining healthy skin and brain functions, facilitating the absorption of iron, and exerting anti-aging effects.

Zinc (energy, digestion)

Magnesium is essential for supporting various bodily functions, including energy production, muscle health, regulation of sleep patterns, digestion, cardiovascular health, and nerve function.

Vitamin C is known for its benefits related to immunity, recuperation, and hormonal balance.

Vitamin D plays a crucial role in regulating the levels of calcium and phosphorus in the body.

Vitamin B12 is essential for energy production, regulation of metabolism, and maintaining a stable mood.

Selenium (fights disease)

Omega-3, known for its beneficial effects on energy levels, heart health, joint health, and skin health

There appears to be a consensus regarding which products either pose hazards or are not deemed worthwhile:
"

Adverse Effects Associated with Testosterone Enhancers (extensive range of undesired outcomes)

Weight gain supplements (the advantages are subject to debate; many of them contain high levels of sugar, artificial sweeteners, and an unfavorable proportion of saturated fats)

HBM (beta-hydroxy beta-methyl butyric acid) exhibits limited efficacy or benefit as a dietary supplement.

The body does not undergo metabolic processes involving glutamine.

L-Arginine has the potential to be neurotoxic and may interact negatively with numerous medications.

Betaine is associated with the occurrence of headaches, herpes outbreaks, and gout.

DMAA, also known as methylhexanamine or dimethylamylamine, constricts blood vessels and concurrently raises blood pressure. This may result in the manifestation of migraines, respiratory distress, constriction of the chest, and potentially even myocardial infarctions.

DMAA has been prohibited from being incorporated into any dietary supplements across Canada.

Synephrine, while potentially hazardous when combined with caffeine, frequently manifests in dietary supplements that include caffeine.

The use of Yohimbe in conjunction with certain medications poses potential hazards.

Additionally, be mindful of the presence of unfavorable substances such as aspartame, artificial dyes, and an excessive amount of caffeine. The incorrect supplements are replete with those ingredients.

The Mechanisms Involved In Muscular Development

Your physique solely recognizes opposition. Your physique is indifferent to whether you're performing a 100-pound bench press or a standard push-up. Your physical constitution lacks the ability to discern between exerting force through the use of six plates on the lat pull down machine, as opposed to performing a customary pull up.

During the process of engaging in resistance training, the muscle fibers in the targeted region undergo a breakdown. For instance, performed a set of 10 repetitions on the preacher curl machine? During the completion of those 10 repetitions, under the condition that you effectively concentrate on the specific engagement of your bicep and establish a strong connection between your mind and muscle, the minute muscle fibers within your bicep are gradually undergoing degradation. After leaving the gym, it is advisable to consume nutritious food and prioritize sound sleep, as this will facilitate the growth and strengthening of the muscles. Capiche? Perform the same process consecutively on each muscle throughout your body.

As previously mentioned, the human body does not differentiate between various types of resistance, but rather recognizes the magnitude of the force exerted upon it. To be unequivocal, I presume that if you are perusing this literary work, you either frequent a fitness facility equipped with weights or possess a personal gymnasium of your own (given that this volume serves as a guide for weightlifting). Achieving a well-toned physique is feasible through bodyweight training and resistance bands. However, if your desired objective is to obtain a sculpted physique characterized by pronounced musculature, a V-shaped torso, prominent trapezius muscles, broad shoulders, and tapered waist, I believe engaging in gym-based exercises will be necessary. Engaging in bodyweight and resistance band exercises can contribute to muscle growth, albeit not to the same magnitude as traditional weightlifting. Increasing the amount of weight you can lift is an essential requirement for developing a robust and sculpted physique, which may not be accomplished to the same degree through bodyweight and resistance training methods.

Developing lean muscle mass, strength, and size requires a gradual and consistent approach. The rate of muscle gain or fat burning greatly depends on the role played by your genetic makeup. Regrettably, one has no dominion over their genetics; however, they do possess authority over their regimen pertaining to exercise, nutrition, and sleep. Hence, we shall focus our attention on these aspects for the time being.

Developing Substantial Muscular Strength Through Implementing These 6 Essential Principles Of Weight Training

In the subsequent segment, I shall establish the foundations pertaining to the core principles of weight training. Please consider the following principles when developing your training program (which we will address subsequently), in order to effectively enhance and develop lean muscle mass.

Compound Movements

Compound exercises are physical activities that engage several primary muscle groups during the movement. These groups offer the most value for your investment. Due to their ability to engage multiple muscle groups simultaneously, these exercises allow for optimal workout efficiency. It is noteworthy that the body's production of growth hormone peaks during the performance of these specific movements, ultimately facilitating optimal muscle bui

Compound movements are exercises such as the bench press, deadlifts, squats, pullups etc. These exercises are specifically designed to target multiple muscle fibers within the major muscle groups, which consequently renders them the most challenging to perform. If your goal is to enhance lean muscle mass, increase strength, and add size to your physique, it is recommended that the majority of your training regimen focuses on compound movements.

Isolation Movements

Isolation movements refer to exercises specifically designed to solely engage and focus on a single muscle group, hence the term "isolation", enabling the targeted isolation of a particular muscle group. While isolation exercises do not simultaneously break down muscle fibers in multiple muscle groups, they indeed aid in effectively targeting and developing specific muscles.

Isolation movements encompass exercises like bicep curls, tricep pull downs, calf raises, preacher curls, among others. These exercises are characterized by their ability to isolate specific muscle groups and are less strenuous compared to compound exercises. From my perspective, the utilization of isolation exercises should be limited to addressing the weaker areas of your physique. If your triceps and calves are areas that could benefit from improvement, engaging in triceps pulldowns and calf raises can assist in enhancing their development to achieve a more balanced and harmonious physique.

Free Weights

These are the weights that elicit activation in your stabilizer muscles upon utilization, specifically referring to dumbbells and barbells. Free weights are highly beneficial for developing structural soundness and enhancing functional strength as they engage the stabilizer muscles.

Although it is possible to lift more weight during a smith machine press in comparison to a barbell bench press, the activation of stabilizer muscles is still lacking in the former. Hence, I propose that the majority of your training program incorporates free weight lifts for the following primary rationale: not only will the utilization of free weights contribute to enhancing your structural integrity and posture, but it will also fortify the stabilizer muscles, thereby augmenting functional strength. Furthermore, engaging in the utilization of ponderous iron free weights exudes a formidable and masculine air, in stark contrast to lifting on a machine. However, it is imperative to note that this standpoint is solely subjective.

Machines

Clearly, machines have their designated purpose; otherwise, their existence would be inconceivable. Perhaps it is just my perspective on technology, but I simply do not have a favorable disposition towards machines. It could be attributed to the fact that my concerns lie in the areas of both building structural integrity and enhancing functional strength, which are aspects that tend to be compromised when utilizing exercise machines.

One can still achieve optimal muscle stimulation through the use of machines; however, it is advisable to exclusively focus on utilizing free weights. Additionally, I would recommend that you make an effort to utilize the exercise equipment available at your nearby fitness facility. Assess the sensation upon your physique, and should you find them more preferable than free weights, disregard my advice and instead prioritize your bodily sensations and personal encounters. If your objective is to develop lean muscle mass, augment your physique, enhance your structural robustness, and heighten your functional strength, then free weights provide the optimal solution. However, if your primary concern is constructing a formidable physique, I am confident that utilizing machines will yield satisfactory results.

Dumbbells

The exercise equipment in question consists of weighted objects attached to a single handle. The dumbbell is highly effective in facilitating profound stretching and contraction during exercises, while also serving to rectify any underlying muscular imbalances one may possess. Based on personal observation, dumbbells have demonstrated a heightened engagement of stabilizer muscles compared to the barbell.

The issue lies in the fact that it is highly probable that your ability to lift with a barbell will be inferior when compared to that with a dumbbell. As an illustration, assume you have a maximal achievable weight of 220 pounds in the barbell bench press exercise. For the majority of individuals, it is unlikely that one would be able to achieve the identical maximum weight lifted for a single repetition using a pair of dumbbells weighing 110 pounds. When transitioning from barbells to dumbbells, there is typically a decline in weight capacity. While the following assertion is based on my personal understanding, it is worth noting that the increased engagement of stabilizer muscles during dumbbell exercises, in comparison to barbell exercises, could be a contributing factor. Additionally, it is possible that certain muscle imbalances, imperceptible during barbell exercises, may also be relevant to this phenomenon.

Barbells

The supreme sovereign of iron. Barbell exercises are highly effective for achieving muscle overload and engaging in high-intensity weightlifting. Barbell exercises are more effective for working the legs as compared to dumbbells. The task of maintaining stability while handling a pair of 110-pound dumbbells is considerably more challenging than squatting with a 220-pound barbell. They are additionally indispensable for performing Olympic lifts such as the clean and jerk or the snatch.

The barbell proves to be effective in achieving muscle overload and facilitating heavier lifts, as it places less emphasis on engaging the stabilizer muscles compared to dumbbells. Nevertheless, the stabilizer muscles are still effectively strengthened during barbell exercises.

Points To Takeaway

When utilizing machines, one may neglect the activation of stabilizer muscles, subsequently compromising their structural integrity and functional strength. Nevertheless, it is possible to attain a higher weight capacity and achieve an effective muscle pump.

When utilizing free weights, although the capacity to lift excessive weight may be limited in comparison to that of a machine, the engagement of your stabilizer muscles contributes significantly to enhancing your overall structural stability. These benefits seamlessly carry over to augment your functional strength.

When utilizing dumbbells, it may be the case that the amount of weight you can lift is less in comparison to a barbell.

Nevertheless, this form of exercise would result in enhanced activation of the stabilizer muscles and the rectification of any existing muscular imbalances that may be present.

Lastly, it should be noted that while barbells may not engage the stabilizer muscles as effectively or address muscular imbalances to the same extent, they still facilitate substantial muscle stimulation and promote effective muscle overload.

Ultimately, I believe that the outcome is contingent upon one's individual inclination. Regardless of whether you derive pleasure from employing machinery or utilizing free weight dumbbells or barbells, the underlying concept remains that of resistance, which entails various pros and cons for each method. Ultimately, employing a blend of all available options is the most advisable course of action. If I were in your position, I would recommend incorporating a combination of barbell, dumbbell, and machines into your training regimen. By exploring and identifying your preferred equipment, you can refine your routine and exclusively focus on that selection.

The Equipment

Whether you possess access to a fitness facility or intend to engage in weightlifting within the confines of your dwelling, we are pleased to furnish you with a comprehensive inventory of equipment that will serve as a foundation as you embark upon your fitness odyssey. Certainly, you possess the fundamental element – your physical being! By leveraging supplementary apparatus, you will amplify your physical capabilities and expedite your progress towards your desired objectives.

Stability Ball

This particular apparatus is known by several distinct designations. Regardless of whether you refer to it as an exercise ball, a stability ball, or a Swiss ball, this piece of equipment is highly effective for focusing on your core muscles. Although the cost of these items may range from $27 to $45, they offer excellent value for the investment. In addition to offering a variety of abdominal exercises, this versatile equipment can serve as a remarkable alternative to a conventional bench when necessary.

Dumbbells and Medicine Balls

If your intention is to engage in weightlifting, it will be necessary to possess a decent collection of dumbbells. We recommend incorporating a diverse range of weights into your workout routine, allowing for progressive weight increments as your strength and capacity improve. It would be beneficial to have various weights at your disposal for targeting different muscle groups. For instance, heavier weights are recommended for performing squats, while lighter weights are advisable for exercising the arms. Regardless, incorporating a high-quality set of dumbbells can expedite the process of building muscle mass compared to solely relying on body weight exercises.

If you do not prefer using dumbbells, you may be familiar with the concept of medicine balls. These weights possess a reduced size and are endowed with additional versatility when compared to dumbbells. As an illustration, these weights are optimal for engaging in core-focused workouts and are available in an extensive range of weight options. Ultimately, what matters most is possessing equipment that brings you satisfaction and facilitates optimal comfort during use.

Resistance Bands

Resistance bands are available in a diverse assortment of resistance levels, dimensions, and widths. For instance, large resistance bands can contribute to the intensification of squats, while smaller bands can aid in targeting smaller muscle groups. Although not indispensable for muscle development, this flexible instrument can prove to be useful on occasions when one chooses to forgo the use of dumbbells.

Workout Mat

If your intention is to engage in home-based exercise, it is advisable to procure a conducive and comfortable environment. A mat can aid in alleviating the discomfort and stress on joints during physical activities. Irrespective of whether you are in a kneeling or reclining position, utilizing a non-slip surface mat can effectively safeguard against potential injuries. They also provide great support for stretching or engaging in relaxation activities such as yoga. Despite the price range typically lying between $16 to $25, they truly warrant the expenditure.

Utilization of Gym & Fitness Equipment and Exercise Tools in a Residential Setting

Experts in the field of bodybuilding acknowledge that this form of training not only enhances your physical appearance but also augments your cognitive abilities. Therefore, we must once again engage our intellect, as there are instances where one may not desire to venture outside, yet it remains essential to maintain physical fitness. The most unfavorable outcome would be the implementation of a lockdown as a consequence of the pandemic. Therefore, it entails more than experiencing an unsettling sensation of reluctance to depart from one's residence. It is possible that working out from home may become a customary practice, therefore what would be the next course of action?

Common equipment such as the Dumbbells and Barbells readily spring to mind, yet prior to embarking on a shopping venture to acquire these indispensable items, have you ensured your familiarity with their proper utilization within a home setting? Do you have all the necessary tools required to shape your physique according to your intended goals?

Initially, it is imperative to ensure that your exercise regimen is harmonized with the requisite equipment pertinent to that specific routine. Subsequently, it is important to take into account the specific area within the residence that you intend to utilize. There are a considerable number of intricacies and specific details to consider when thoroughly examining the matter. Prior to proceeding, it is appropriate to acknowledge those individuals who demonstrate concern for their fellow bodybuilding peers and intend to present them with a fitness accessory.

Discovering the finest wellness presents for your exercise enthusiast coworker or family member has never been easier. When the pandemic necessitated the closure of gyms for an extended duration, individuals were compelled to employ ingenuity in order to maintain their physical fitness. The demand for in-home exercise equipment and accessories experienced an increase. Fitness facilities may have resumed operations. Nevertheless, certain individuals have discovered that engaging in exercise routines in the comfort of their own residences can be inherently enjoyable.

We are currently unaware of the duration for which the gyms will remain open. Nevertheless, there is an infinite array of trinkets that acquaintances who congregate at the fitness center exchange. Moreover, even individuals who genuinely experience a sense of wellness would value these products irrespective of the context in which they are utilized. Nonetheless, the act of presenting a piece of equipment can be quite delicate if one lacks knowledge regarding the individual's preferred practices.

As an illustration, it is incumbent upon you to exclusively consider one specimen from each assortment. A myriad of activities can be performed utilizing one's own body weight and a few exercise apparatus, thereby offering heightened convenience while exercising within the confines of one's residence.

The aim during this time frame is to surpass the limitations we frequently impose on ourselves. Below, you will find a curated selection of top-notch gym equipment, including fitness accessories like jump ropes, kettlebells, gloves, and hats, all of which will greatly enhance your loved one's workout sessions.

Jump Rope

During my formative years, I frequently engaged in double dutch skipping with my cousins, rendering the activity devoid of its intended physical exertion. Regardless, to my utter astonishment, the act of using a skipping rope has been shown to effectively strengthen both the upper and lower extremities. After a short series of jumps, the sensation will start to manifest in your lower extremities. It currently stands as a primary enhancer of endurance and resilience. To elevate the intensity of the exercises, one may incorporate a weighted rope to enhance the strength and conditioning of the muscles in the shoulders and chest region. I would gladly choose a youth play as an activity without hesitation, no matter the time or day. Additionally, it serves as an exceptional fitness apparatus.

Dumbbells

These items epitomize the venerable cornerstone of the bodybuilder's gym, as they can be employed in a myriad of ways. They are also one of the limited fitness equipment options available in the exercise facility, yet they are equally proficient when utilized at home. Dumbbells are cherished by numerous trainers as they afford the opportunity to enhance overall body development, a factor of utmost importance to us. Irrespective of the necessity to engage the lower extremities and assume a squatting position, dumbbells can effectively target nearly every muscle group, including augmenting arm strength through bicep curls. This tool is highly regarded for its beneficial effects on wellness, making it an ideal choice for professional trainers seeking a convenient and effective addition to their home or preferred training environments.

Kettlebells

In juxtaposition to dumbbells, the distribution of weight in the kettlebell is not evenly spread. This suggests that a greater level of physical strength and adaptation is required to effectively manage one's body and weight during the practice of kettlebell exercises. There is no specific body part designated for practice with this. You have the capacity to engage in fundamental exercises targeting the core, upper body, particularly arms and back, and even lower body. The kettlebell offers myriad creative possibilities. They are available in a range of loads, allowing you to choose the most suitable option based on your individual strength capabilities.

Exercise Bands for Toning and Strengthening

There exists a wide array of "resistance bands," each of which serves different purposes and is employed distinctively. These specific groups are commonly referred to as "booty bands" due to their vital role in conditioning and developing the gluteal muscles. By providing resistance to movements such as donkey kicks, hip bridges, jumping squats, and other exercises targeting the glutes, these bands prompt the muscles to exert greater effort. The bars are available in three levels of resistance, namely light, medium, and heavy, catering to individuals at different wellness levels. Whilst certain variations are produced using a textile similar to elastic bands, they have a tendency to ascend along the thighs and potentially hinder physical activity, particularly for individuals with more substantial thigh proportions.

Yoga Mats

Even if you are not attending conventional yoga classes, it should not deter you from practicing yoga regularly. Yoga mats provide a cushioned surface for your body during physical activities, be it performing yoga postures or engaging in abdominal exercises. Exercising with the mat can enhance your stability due to its surface grip, which helps protect against injuries and creates a safe and steady environment for your workouts. The best part? Mats can typically be relocated and neatly positioned in a corner after use to ensure minimal disruption. They have no intention of doing so! In fact, you could even opt to strategically position your dumbbells down the center in order to achieve a much larger space-saving outcome.

Pharmaceutical Slam Spheres

Indeed, it is quite probable that you believe there are limited possibilities when it comes to utilizing a weighted slam ball. Nevertheless, I assure you that the possibilities are limitless. I became familiar with medicine balls at the gym and promptly identified a variety of exercises that can be performed with this equipment. A multitude of physical movements can also serve as comprehensive exercises for the entire body. This particular choice is highly regarded by individuals who possess a deep understanding of its concealed intricacies. Exceptionally suitable for rigorous cardiovascular workouts, as they effectively maintain an elevated heart rate. This exercise strengthens the abdominal muscles and engages the entire chest region, simultaneously involving the lower body when executing leg movements between repetitions. Envision a solitary apparatus, effectively providing a comprehensive workout for the entire body.

Extended Elastic Straps

In contrast to booty bands, the development of elongated resistance bands specifically formulated to facilitate comprehensive physical workouts has taken place. These remarkable stretchable fasteners may not appear intimidating. Nevertheless, they prove to be strenuous tasks. The potential possibilities are immeasurable with these. Your musculature can be strengthened through a range of exercises. One can seamlessly transition from executing posterior column exercises to performing shoulder presses, all the while experiencing comparable resistance from the band without the burden of dumbbells. The weight of the band undergoes a transformation through the use of shading. Nevertheless, it is undeniable that they can be interconnected to support substantially greater amounts of weight. An advantageous feature of these is their ability to be shared with entryways, enabling additional workouts that would typically be performed at a fitness facility.

Gliding Disks

These diminutive circular discs bear resemblance to a frisbee. Nevertheless, they are not employed for such purposes of amusement. These disks are employed for the purpose of facilitating a seamless sliding surface for the feet and hands during exercise. These exercises have been specifically formulated to target and correct your core as you engage in the motions. Some of my preferred exercises, with these being hikers and side lunges.

Cones

It is widely believed that the use of cones requires a certain level of creativity; nonetheless, they serve as a valuable asset to any workout regimen when a proper routine is established. Cone exercises are renowned in sports such as football for the purpose of developing speed and agility through structured drills. During physical training sessions, these exercises can effectively enhance muscular strength and promote agility through alternative means.

Ab Rollers

Hello, core, please smile for the camera! Possessing a strong core can offer benefits across multiple domains, encompassing enhanced equilibrium and refined posture. Simply incorporate the ab roller into your exercise routine. It appears to be a fundamentally rudimentary tool - precisely, a handle with grips - however, its fabrication can be exceedingly demanding. Performing a few repetitions of wheel rollouts while assuming a kneeling position will induce abdominal muscle soreness, ultimately resulting in enhanced core strength and resilience.

Massage Guns

Engaging in bodybuilding can provide immense enjoyment and gratification, until one awakens the next day to find their muscles noticeably fatigued and tender as a result of the demanding workout undertaken the previous day. While Epsom salt baths can provide considerable relief from this discomfort, a specialized tool designed specifically for this purpose exists: introducing, the massage device. The invigorating performance of this product plays a pivotal role in ensuring that muscles receive the proper care they deserve after exercise. The versatility of a Theragun is truly a godsend.

Weighted Bands for the Ankles and Wrists

If you are in pursuit of lightweight equipment that will incorporate a slight element of resistance into your daily routine, then the 'Ankle or wrist weights' serve as an exceptional choice. These portable burdens afford the wearer unrestricted mobility, and they facilitate a rigorous workout.

The Database Method

It is a challenging task to browse through Instagram without encountering a video featuring someone engaged in the act of construction. This versatile apparatus has become one of my preferred choices, given the closure of the fitness center. The velocity is remarkable, as is its potency. Furthermore, a myriad of activities beyond the stimulation of the gluteus maximus can be undertaken with these tools. Fitness equipment endorsed by the Kardashian family, offering the convenience of a 10-minute high-intensity workout while also facilitating a comprehensive exercise routine. Nevertheless, the weighted seat provides diverse exercises that engage the abdominal muscles, obliques, and arms.

Furthermore, we must not overlook the embellishments, as they possess utmost charm and appeal. The DB Method 10lb belt facilitates a seamless transition between a range of exercises, including jumping jacks and lunges. In fact, it has become an integral part of my exercise routine, to the point that I do not engage in physical activity without it. Although this may entail a substantial investment, the accompanying features of the machine are truly remarkable and contribute to a truly pleasurable experience.

Peloton Bike

If you have a great passion for cycling, then the Peloton bicycle was specifically crafted with individuals like you in mind. The monthly membership option for cycling is an excellent choice for individuals who have a deep passion for pedaling. Additionally, cycling is exceptional for the remarkable cardiovascular and muscular endurance it entails. The Peloton bicycle can also provide an immersive experience, simulating the feeling of working out alongside comrades through its interactive live classes conducted online. The bike is expensive. Nevertheless, it can be settled through incremental and scheduled disbursements. Assuming all factors are constant, after the expenses incurred for cycling classes, the resultant cost can be roughly equivalent.

Headphones

To be honest, it is not uncommon for individuals to choose to forgo a physical activity due to the mere oversight of forgetting to bring their headphones. Indeed, although it may seem rather frivolous, music possesses the capacity to serve as substantial motivation to persevere through a rigorous exercise regimen. Several individuals may find that a pair of earphones is the preferred gadget for promoting daydreaming and concentration during physical activity. If you happen to belong to this category of individuals, there is no need for any discomfort or awkwardness. Provided that the task is completed. Telecommuting entails various disruptions, however, by donning your headphones and increasing the volume of the music, you establish the rhythm for the subsequent 30 minutes, hour, or whichever duration your schedule dictates.

Supplements

For individuals who prioritize their health and value their supplements just as much as their exercise equipment, surprising them with the replenishment of their favorite products would be a thoughtful gift. Offer a gift that will provide a boost to a friend's workout routine, ranging from nutrient-rich blends to pre-exercise supplements.

General accessories

In terms of exercise accessories, there is a wide array of items that your companion may necessitate. Make necessary arrangements for protective gloves to be readily available, serving the dual purpose of safeguarding their hands and providing a barrier against germs. Additionally, provide a duffle sack for each individual to securely store their personal belongings. A cap is considered a prominent accessory by the bodybuilder. During days when the hair looks particularly unappealing, it becomes an indispensable requirement. Certain individuals have a distinct preference for Top Knot caps due to the thoughtful design of their perspiration wick material, which includes appealing finishes that enable the wearer to fashion their hair into elevated pigtails and buns during exercise.

How To Develop An Effective Weight Loss Program

First and foremost, it is imperative to cultivate a comprehension of the physiological mechanisms associated with elevated levels of adipose tissue. Consider the factors contributing to adipose accumulation in distinct anatomical regions, and reflect upon the potential ramifications this may have on our overall well-being. It is imperative to comprehend certain technical terminologies and behavioral patterns associated with weight gain.

Energy

Energy is derived from the sun and is referred to as "light energy." Through the mechanism of photosynthesis, plants transform light energy into a stored chemical energy. Subsequently, we obtain the requisite energy through the consumption of these plants or via animal sources that partake in the consumption of said plants.

Energy is accumulated within our nourishment in the structures of lipid, protein, and carbohydrate compounds. These represent the primary macronutrients that undergo breakdown processes to provide the body with energy, subsequently utilized by the organism.

Energy is distributed and employed in various undertakings, serving the purpose of constructing muscle and facilitating the revitalization of impaired tissue subsequent to physical exertion or trauma. Additionally, it is employed for conveying various substances such as glucose, which serves as the primary fuel for our bodies, as well as calcium, to cell membranes. A marginal quantity of energy is expended to sustain skeletal muscle activity, enabling the body to facilitate locomotion and produce mechanical power.

The muscular activity significantly imposes strain on the body's capacity to generate energy, considering that during vigorous physical exertion, like sprinting, the energy expenditure can surpass that needed during rest by a magnitude of a thousand.

Macronutrients

As previously mentioned, macronutrients serve as the primary sources of energy for our bodies and encompass fat, protein, and carbohydrate. Fat has a caloric value of 9.3 kilocalories per gram. Protein exhibits an energy yield of 4.3 kcal per gram, while carbohydrates possess an energy yield of 4.1 kcal per gram.

A modest quantity of adipose tissue is essential for the proper functioning of our bodies, notwithstanding the prevalent belief that adiposity is detrimental and detrimental to our overall well-being. Nevertheless, it represents a considerable reservoir of energy, with a mere 1kg of stored body fat being capable of providing a substantial 7,000 kcals of energy.

Even individuals possessing a notably slender physique have the capacity to depend on their adipose reserves for the purpose of fueling their bodily functions. The human body possesses a considerable reservoir of stored energy in the form of fat, which has the potential to be utilized as a source of energy. For instance, an individual who falls within the average weight range and maintains a body fat percentage of approximately 13% has the capacity to store approximately 70,000 kilocalories (kcals) of fat, a sufficient amount to sustain a distance of 1,126 kilometers. Their carbohydrate reserves would amount to approximately. 2,500 kilocalories, an amount of energy that corresponds to the caloric expenditure needed to complete a 40 kilometer run.

The adipose tissue surrounding our internal organs serves as insulation, providing warmth and acting as a reservoir of energy for later utilization. These aforementioned factors represent only a subset of the numerous rationales behind the accumulation of adipose tissue in our bodies.

Adipose tissue is partitioned into two distinct compartments – adipose depots and essential fat.

Storage fat primarily consists of adipose tissue, encompassing both subcutaneous fat and visceral fat which serves to safeguard the internal organs in the thoracic and abdominal cavity against injuries.

Vital adipose tissue is distributed and deposited throughout various regions of the body, encompassing lipid-rich tissues within our central nervous system, heart, lungs, kidneys, liver, intestines, spleen, in addition to bone marrow and muscles.

Essential fat is needed for normal physiological functioning. Females possess distinct sex-related essential fat deposits in areas such as the buttocks, thighs, pelvis, and breasts, which serve pivotal roles in both reproductive capabilities and hormonal regulation.

Despite the ongoing discussions, it has been established that both males and females possess a comparable level of fat storage. The percentage of fat storage in males is approximately 12%, while in females it is around 15%. Moreover, it is noteworthy that the overall essential fat percentage in females, which encompasses sex-specific fat, exceeds the utility of essential fat in males by a factor of approximately four.

The human body accumulates fatty substances within specialized cells called adipocytes or fat cells, which are specifically designed to store energy in the form of fat. The adipose tissue comprises triglycerides, which can be hydrolyzed to provide a source of energy. The cells function to store surplus fats and facilitate their accessibility for utilization during periods of energy demand.

An individual of average weight typically possesses approximately 25-30 billion adipocytes, whereas an obese individual may possess an elevated number ranging from 42-106 billion. The average dimensions of adipocytes in an individual with obesity are approximately 40% greater in comparison to those of an individual with a healthy body weight.

A significant portion of our body fat is stored within adipose tissue, which primarily comprises approximately 83% fat, accompanied by supportive structures consisting of roughly 15% water and 2% protein.

Adipose tissue is characterized by two specific subtypes: white adipose tissue (WAT), responsible for storage of fat, and brown adipose tissue (BAT), involved in heat production.

Brown adipose tissue is commonly denominated as fetal adipose tissue, as it primarily exists in neonates and fulfills the role of generating thermal energy essential for the neonate's sustenance.

As adults, if we experience increments in body weight due to overeating, our pre-existing adipocytes gradually accumulate additional lipids, leading to an enlargement in size. This phenomenon is commonly referred to as hypertrophy of adipose cells.

When an individual classified as obese experiences significant weight gain, they will ultimately reach a stage referred to as 'maturity onset severe obesity,' where there is further accumulation of body fat. The adipocytes eventually reach a state of hypertrophy beyond which they are unable to further expand their size. As

173

adipocytes reach their maximum size, the cumulative number of these cells grows through a phenomenon referred to as "fat cell hyperplasia." It is widely posited that the adiposity level of individuals classified as obese, approximately equivalent to 170% of the average body weight, typically amounts to roughly 60%. It is after this point that a notable correlation between adipocyte proliferation and an escalation in the number of adipocytes can be observed.

Upon an individual's weight loss, the adipocyte cells of each person decrease in size, without any alteration in their quantity or location, as they await replenishment.

Typically, it is customary for individuals to accumulate adipose tissue primarily in the abdominal region or thighs. Let us now explore the factors responsible for variations in the distribution of body fat across specific regions of the human body.

Lipoprotein lipase serves as an enzymatic catalyst for the process of facilitating the absorption and storage of triglycerides within adipocytes. The diverse range of lipoprotein activity plays a pivotal role in the variance of fat distribution among individuals and exerts an influence on the alterations in fat distribution that occur during middle age and pregnancy.

The disparity in the distribution of total body fat between genders can be attributed to the greater concentration of lipoprotein found in females. In women, substantial quantities of lipoprotein are produced by the adipocytes in the breast, thigh, and hip regions. In contrast, in males, it is the abdominal fat cells that demonstrate activity with the lipoprotein enzyme.

In the context of weight loss in obese individuals, the reduction in body weight prompts an elevation in lipoprotein levels within their fat cells, consequently facilitating the potential for weight and body fat restoration. The greater the initial body size and level of obesity prior to weight loss, the more determinedly the body will endeavor to reacquire the lost weight.

Gynoid obesity, also known as pear-shaped body, refers to a body type characterized by an accumulation of adipose tissue in the hips and thighs.

Android obesity tends to be predominantly prevalent among males, wherein the body shape often exhibits an apple-like appearance, with a greater concentration of adipose tissue around the abdominal region and upper body. This phenomenon typically exposes individuals to a heightened susceptibility to type 2 diabetes, hypertension, hypercholesterolemia, coronary heart disease, various forms of cancer, and untimely mortality as opposed to individuals with gynoid obesity.

Excessive adiposity can have detrimental effects on one's overall well-being, and the distribution of adipose tissue holds significance in this context. The potential negative health implications for individuals with android obesity surpass those observed in individuals with gynoid obesity. This is due to the fact that, metabolically, the abdomen exhibits a higher level of responsiveness in comparison to the adipose tissue stored in the thighs and hips. As a consequence, it is more prone to breaking down, ultimately resulting in the development of atherosclerosis, heart disease, and various other severe ailments.

While it is commonly observed that android obesity tends to affect men more frequently, and gynoid obesity tends to affect women, it is worth noting that there are cases where men experience gynoid obesity and vice versa.

The Causes of Obesity

According to reports in Britain, it is projected that by the year 2050, a significant portion of our population will experience a predominance of obesity, with an estimated 60% of men and 50% of women classified as clinically obese.

Numerous individuals often attribute their weight gain to genetics and hormone issues; however, empirical evidence indicates that the primary driver of the escalating obesity rates is mostly a culmination of unhealthy dietary habits and sedentary lifestyles. The etiology of obesity is multifaceted, encompassing diverse factors that intricately influence an individual's susceptibility to excessive weight gain.

The many factors include:

Genetics

Energy imbalance

Hormonal imbalance

Conditions pertaining to trauma, emotional, and psychological disturbances

The impact of cultural factors and surrounding conditions

The primary factor contributing to obesity among the aforementioned factors is an imbalance of energy.

Energy equilibrium is commonly referred to as:

The energy derived from food is equivalent to the energy expended, resulting in the maintenance of body fat stores at a constant level.

In the event that the amount of energy you consume surpasses the amount of energy you exert, an energy imbalance ensues, and consequently, the surplus energy is deposited as adipose tissue.

Approximately equals one kilogram of body fat. An excess of 7,000 calories of untapped energy. For this reason, even a slight energy imbalance can have a significant impact on long-term weight gain.

According to scholarly research and empirical data, it is evident that the primary factors contributing to the surge in obesity and weight gain can be attributed to the convergence of shifts in dietary habits and a sedentary way of life.

Individuals who utilize lesser amounts of energy compared to others tend to lead less physically active lifestyles, in conjunction with consuming excessive amounts of energy-dense convenience foods that are rich in fat. This combination ultimately gives rise to an imbalance in energy levels.

Over the past two decades in the United Kingdom, research studies have revealed that the primary factors contributing to the rise in body weight among the average male and female population are characterized by an upsurge in overall energy consumption coupled with a decline in physical activity levels, affecting both genders. The primary factor contributing to weight gain was the rise in energy consumption.

The nourishment and beverages we intake afford us with vitality. The inclusion of calorie-dense and nutrient-poor foods, characterized by high levels of sugar and fat, in our dietary intake is a common occurrence. Such foods, devoid of significant vitamins, minerals, and other micronutrients, fail to provide essential nutrients necessary for maintaining good health. Instead, they solely contribute to weight gain, thereby exacerbating various health issues in the long run.

Research indicates that individuals with obesity tend to consume fewer calories compared to their counterparts of similar age and gender who maintain average body fat percentages, yet exhibit significantly lower levels of physical activity.

Insufficient physical exertion leads to an increase in body weight. Some factors that have contributed to the decrease in physical activity include the proliferation of labor-saving devices, such as elevators and escalators, the decline in manual labor jobs, and the growing popularity of sedentary activities such as computer games, to mention only a few examples.

The maintenance of energy equilibrium, commonly referred to as energy balance, occurs when the caloric intake matches the energy expenditure, thereby preventing significant alterations in the body's fat reserves. When there is a discrepancy between the amount of energy consumed and the amount of energy expended, this leads to an energy imbalance resulting in the accumulation of surplus energy in the form of adipose tissue.

The degree of energy imbalance may differ among individuals due to a combination of genetic tendencies, individual behavior, and environmental influences.

The development of obesity in children with obese parents may be attributed to their lifestyle choices rather than their genetic predisposition.

Obesity-associated genetic factors may exert an influence on the allocation of body adipose tissue in the subsequent manner:

Certain genes have the potential to decrease the likelihood of engaging in physical exercise, as they possess the ability to influence our body's food metabolism and fat storage mechanisms. If a child possesses a sole parent characterized by obesity, their likelihood of developing obesity is already at 40%. It has the potential to influence behavior, leading us to adopt unfavorable lifestyle habits that promote an increased likelihood of experiencing obesity. Genetic factors can enhance our sensitivity to the visual, olfactory, and gustatory aspects of food, potentially influencing our taste perception. Consequently, these genetic variations may contribute to a preference for foods rich in unhealthy fats, while also leading to a reduced inclination towards the flavors of nutritious organic foods. Finally, the influence of genetic factors can impact and regulate our appetite to an extent that it impedes our ability to perceive satiety.

The environment also exerts a significant influence:

An Inactive Lifestyle - Western societies characterized by individuals leading increasingly sedentary lives have a pronounced impact on the prevalence of obesity. Overdependence on technology further leads to a reduction in energy expenditure and diminished levels of physical activity.

Automobile utilization – the utilization of automobiles has shown a consistent upward trend, with an increasing number of individuals opting to remain indoors due to apprehensions regarding safety and criminal activities. There has been a noticeable decline in the number of children utilizing buses in recent times, with a growing proportion of parents opting to personally transport their children to school rather than allowing them to commute on foot.

Lifestyle & Convenience – It remains feasible to develop obesity, even in the absence of a genetic inclination. The sedentary nature and elevated stress levels within our environment have contributed to the convenient availability of reasonably priced, high-fat food options. Opting for taste and convenience presents a more accessible choice.

The environment plays a significant role in reducing the likelihood of engaging in physical activity, as individuals often feel uneasy utilizing urban streets. The worsening conditions for pedestrians have intensified this discomfort, leading people to fear acts of anti-social behavior and crime. Consequently, this apprehension serves as a deterrent to walking and other forms of exercise.

sedentary pastimes such as browsing the internet, playing video games, and watching television, all of which enjoy widespread popularity. An increasing number of individuals are dedicating their time to operating computers, coinciding with the unprecedented popularity of social media platforms.

There are several alternative factors contributing to obesity, encompassing instances such as cerebral trauma or tumors affecting the central mechanisms responsible for hunger, satiety, and energy regulation. Such conditions can lead to varying degrees of obesity.

Even in times when we do not experience hunger, we may still engage in eating as a means to cope with our emotions or alleviate undesirable feelings. In instances of sadness, loneliness, guilt, worry, and boredom, we may resort to using food as a mechanism to overcome these emotional states.

Feelings of inferiority, self-doubt, and the confrontation of fears and challenges contribute to our tendency to overindulge in food.

Management of Body Fat Storage

When the amount of energy consumed is greater than the amount of energy expended, the surplus energy is converted into adipose tissue and stored in the body.

In order to reduce the levels of excessive body fat, it is necessary to establish a negative energy equilibrium by expending more energy than you consume. In order to achieve weight loss, it is necessary to establish an imbalance in energy levels.

For example:

The consumption of energy surpassing the expenditure of energy results in the accumulation of body fat.

Energy in